Treatment of cancer cachexia

Filippo Rossi Fanelli - Maurizio Muscaritoli

Treatment of cancer cachexia

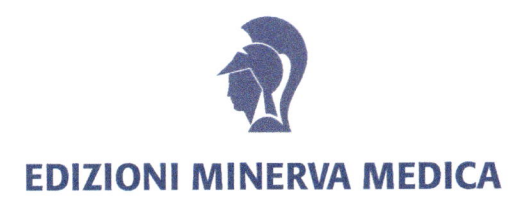

EDIZIONI MINERVA MEDICA

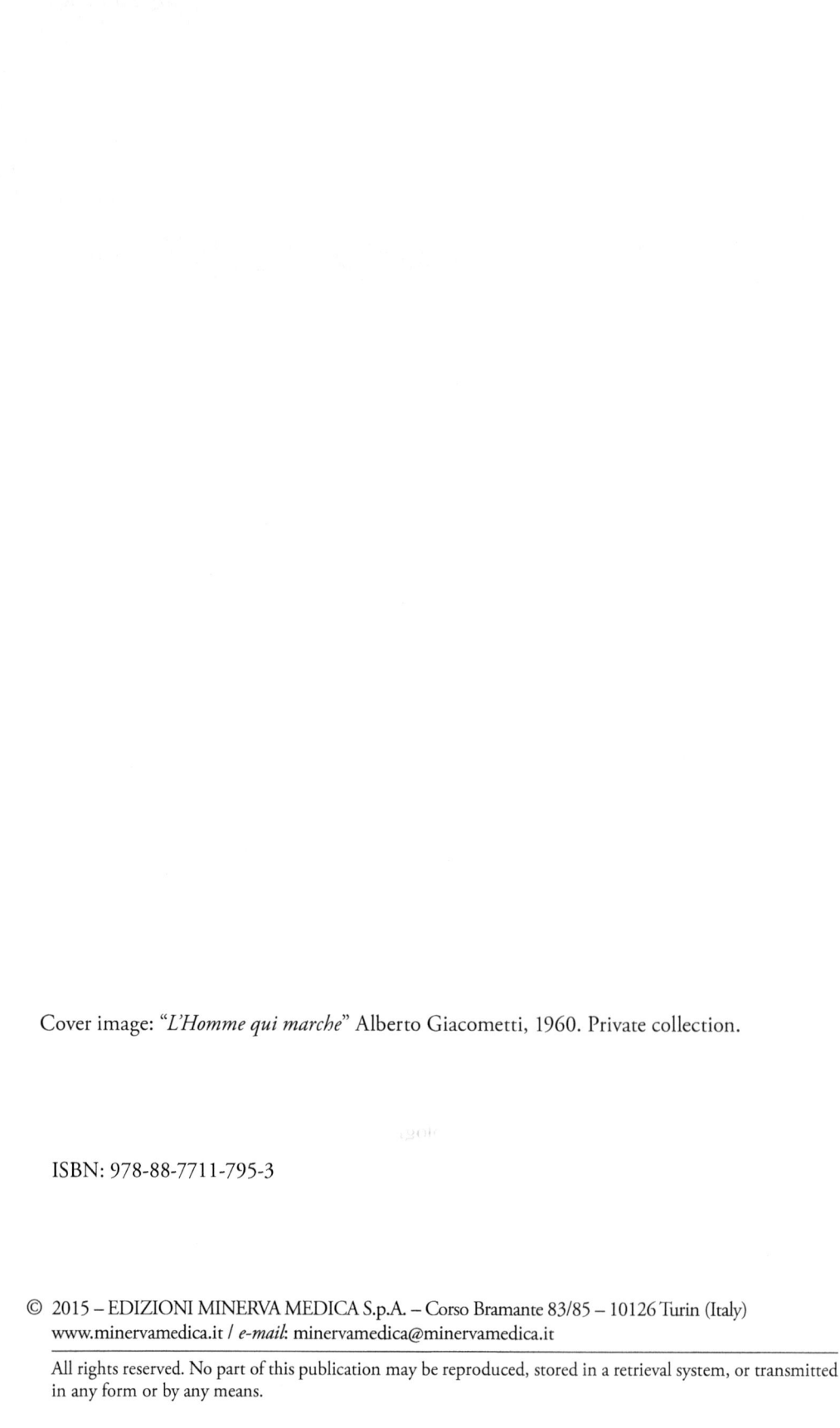

Cover image: "*L'Homme qui marche*" Alberto Giacometti, 1960. Private collection.

ISBN: 978-88-7711-795-3

© 2015 – EDIZIONI MINERVA MEDICA S.p.A. – Corso Bramante 83/85 – 10126 Turin (Italy)
www.minervamedica.it / *e-mail*: minervamedica@minervamedica.it

All rights reserved. No part of this publication may be reproduced, stored in a retrieval system, or transmitted in any form or by any means.

Preface

The incidence of cachexia is of crucial importance for survival in chronic diseases, including cancer. Modern medicine has to deal with this important interdisciplinary problem, worldwide. Cancer is now better treated by novel therapies. New therapeutic strategies represent an advantage over the previous standards of care, but patients continue to face the nutritional and metabolic consequences of the illness process itself and the effects related to the therapies.

This book focuses on cachexia as a clinical syndrome that accompanies different types of cancer. There is not yet an unified definition of cancer cachexia. It may be considered the result of a complex cascade of events including chronic inflammation, free radical generation, chronic hyperactivation of immune and endocrine systems with consequent dysregulation of appetite, hormone resistance syndromes, increased catabolism and impaired anabolism. During recent years research has particularly focused on the role of inflammation and on the dysregulation of most of the catabolic and anabolic pathways. The results of such intensive research should lead in the near future to the development of new treatments for cancer cachexia.

The main signs and symptoms of cachexia are represented by weight loss, muscle and adipose tissue wasting, inflammation, asthenia and loss of appetite. They are often under-recognized in clinical practice.

This book aims to increase awareness of cancer-related metabolic and nutritional impairments, as well as knowledge of the pathophysiological mechanisms of cachexia leading to muscle and fat tissue wasting. The clinical consequences of cachexia are now receiving more attention from health-related professionals as a consequence of the enormous efforts of scientific societies, individual researchers, patient associations, and pharmaceutical industries. Cancer cachexia is an extremely complex syndrome and an important clinical event, particularly because of its implications in terms of increased morbidity, mortality, socio-economic issues and its negative impact on the quality of life.

In summary, cachexia can be analyzed from different perspectives, including those of morphologists, epidemiologists, biochemists, biologists, physiologists, and clinicians. The primary purpose of this work is to spread knowledge of cancer cachexia among health care professionals, and in particular, nutritionists, internists, oncologists and dietitians.

We hope that this book will help to more clearly understand the clinical impact of cancer cachexia, highlighting the importance of the early diagnosis and treatment of this severe and disabling clinical condition.

FILIPPO ROSSI FANELLI

Authors

ZAIRA AVERSA
Department of Clinical Medicine, Sapienza University of Rome, Rome, Italy

PAOLA COSTELLI
Department of Clinical and Biological Sciences, University of Turin, Turin, Italy

GIANFRANCO GIOIA
Department of Clinical Medicine, Sapienza University of Rome, Rome, Italy

ALESSANDRO LAVIANO
Department of Clinical Medicine, Sapienza University of Rome, Rome, Italy

SIMONE LUCIA
Department of Clinical Medicine, Sapienza University of Rome, Rome, Italy

ALESSIA MARI
Department of Clinical Medicine, Sapienza University of Rome, Rome, Italy

ALESSIO MOLFINO
Department of Clinical Medicine, Sapienza University of Rome, Rome, Italy

MAURIZIO MUSCARITOLI
Department of Clinical Medicine, Sapienza University of Rome, Rome, Italy

SERENA RIANDA
Department of Clinical Medicine, Sapienza University of Rome, Rome, Italy

FILIPPO ROSSI FANELLI
Department of Clinical Medicine, Sapienza University of Rome, Rome, Italy

Contents

Preface V
F. Rossi Fanelli

Authors VII

1 **DEFINITION AND CLINICAL FEATURES OF CANCER CACHEXIA** 1
   M. Muscaritoli, S. Lucia, F. Rossi Fanelli

2 **IMPACT OF CANCER CACHEXIA ON PATIENT OUTCOME** 5
   S. Lucia, M. Muscaritoli

3 **BIOCHEMICAL FEATURES OF MUSCLE WASTING IN CANCER CACHEXIA** 11
   P. Costelli, Z. Aversa

4 **ANOREXIA, REDUCED FOOD INTAKE AND SICKNESS BEHAVIOR
   IN CANCER CACHEXIA** 23
   A. Molfino, G. Gioia, A. Laviano

5 **PHARMACOLOGIC THERAPY OF CACHEXIA** 29
   A. Laviano, S. Rianda, A. Mari

6 **NUTRACEUTICALS IN CANCER PATIENTS WITH CACHEXIA** 39
   A. Molfino, G. Gioia

7 **PERSPECTIVES** 45
   F. Rossi Fanelli

DEFINITION AND CLINICAL FEATURES OF CANCER CACHEXIA

M. MUSCARITOLI, S. LUCIA, F. ROSSI FANELLI

Cachexia is a complex and multifactorial syndrome featuring the loss of skeletal muscle mass (with or without loss of fat mass), impairing the quality of life (QoL), and increasing morbidity and mortality in patients affected by chronic diseases. The term "cachexia", derived from the Greek words *kakòs* (bad) and *hexis* (condition or appearance), is associated with a progressive wasting syndrome leading to death. Cachexia originates from the complex interplay between a tumor, host metabolism, and proinflammatory cytokines; it is not fully reversible by conventional nutrition support and it should be differentiated from starvation, age-related loss of muscle mass, primary depression, malabsorption, and hyperthyroidism.[1, 2] Among cancer patients, cachexia accounts for up to 20% to 30% of patient deaths and it is estimated that two million people die annually across the world, solely because of the consequences of cancer-related cachexia.[1, 2] Cancer cachexia has a higher prevalence in gastrointestinal, lung, and head-neck tumors than in other kinds of neoplasia such as breast, hematologic, and endocrine tumors.[3] Until recently, cancer cachexia was considered a terminal cancer event substantially refractory to available treatments and uniquely amenable to palliative support. Currently, a better understanding of its pathogenesis suggests that cachexia should be considered an early phenomenon. Indeed, significant biochemical and molecular changes occur in cancer patients before any evidence of body weight loss, thus suggesting the use of early, appropriate, tailored interventions aimed at preventing, reversing, or delaying the metabolic perturbations that ultimately lead to cachexia. A panel of experts has suggested a multimodal intervention performed by a synergistic approach implemented by oncologists and nutritionists and represented by the so called "parallel pathway".[2] This intervention consists of an early assessment combined with an intensive nutritional and functional follow-up, proceeding in parallel to the oncological follow-up. The scientific community has been focusing on spreading the message that cancer cachexia is not related to the last period of cancer disease, but that it may instead be present from the early phases, even without obvious clinical manifestations: the early detection of cancer cachexia along with a periodic follow-up of nutritional status changes may be an efficacious intervention to treat this devastating condition and even to prevent it.[2] This strategy appears decisive in order to guarantee the patient's best performance during anticancer treatments, thus avoiding administration of scheduled dose reduction or even premature treatment suspension.

Although the pathway is clearly defined, daily practice describes a different scenario: many patients are evaluated too late, when a high percentage of body weight has already been lost and the refractory stage of cancer cachexia has already occurred, rendering available interventions ineffective.

In this light, some authors have recently proposed a classification system and practical diagnostic criteria in order to promote the early detection of cancer cachexia, thus allowing prompt efficacious intervention.[2, 4] Considering cancer cachexia as a continuum, experts have identified three stages of clinical

TREATMENT OF CANCER CACHEXIA

Table 1-I – The main clinical determinants characterizing cancer cachexia staging according to the definition.[4]

	Pre-cachexia	Cachexia	Refractory cachexia
Weight loss	X	X	X
Low BMI		X	
Inflammation	X		
Anorexia	X		
Sarcopenia		X	
Anticancer therapy unresponsiveness			X
Low PS			X
Life expectancy <3 Mo			X

Abbreviations: BMI = Body mass index; PS = Performance status; Mo = Months.

relevance: pre-cachexia, cachexia, and refractory cachexia, distinguishable from each other by different clinical determinants (Tab. 1-I).
- *Pre-cachexia* is defined by unintentional weight loss of ≤5% of usual body weight during the last six months, chronic or recurrent systemic inflammatory response (e.g., elevated serum levels of C-reactive protein), and anorexia or anorexia-related symptoms.
- Patients are classified as having *cachexia* when they have more than 5% loss of stable body weight over the past 6 months, a body-mass index (BMI) less than 20 kg/m² and ongoing weight loss of more than 2%, or sarcopenia and ongoing weight loss of more than 2%.
- In *refractory cachexia*, the cachexia can be clinically refractory as a result of very advanced cancer (pre-terminal) or the presence of rapidly progressive cancer unresponsive to anticancer therapy. This stage is characterized by a low performance status and a life expectancy of less than three months and is associated with active catabolism, or the presence of factors that render the active management of weight loss no longer possible or appropriate.

CLINICAL FEATURES OF CANCER CACHEXIA

Patients with cancer might present with malnutrition (secondary to anorexia and starvation), cachexia, or both. Cachexia should also be differentiated from starvation, age-related loss of muscle mass, primary depression, malabsorption and hyperthyroidism,[5] and should instead be considered a metabolic derangement, originating from the complex interplay between chronic disease, host metabolism and the imbalance between pro-inflammatory and anti-inflammatory cytokines. This interaction also implies an abnormal production of neuropeptides and hormones, at least in part responsible for anorexia, insulin resistance, and increased lipolysis and lipid oxidation, increased protein turnover.[5] Although cachexia is not fully reversible by conventional nutrition support, reduced nutrient availability (because of reduced intake, impaired absorption or increased losses, or a combination of these)[2] may be a significant component and play a role in the pathogenesis of cachexia. Indeed, it is noteworthy that while not all malnourished patients are cachectic, all cachectic patients are invariably malnourished.

The most clinically relevant phenotypic features of cachexia are represented by anorexia, weight loss, inflammation, body composition derangement and sarcopenia.

Chemosensory alterations in cancer and during cancer therapy are well documented,[6] with alterations in taste and smell often contributing to the development of food aversion and reduced hedonic response. The disruption of central and peripheral signaling for regulation of eating behavior in cancer patients may lead to anorexia, defined as the loss of desire to eat, consisting of appetite loss, early satiety and/or altered food behavior finally determining a reduced energy intake.[7, 8] Anorexia accounts for up to 55% of patients at the point of the cancer diagnosis and this is even higher in terminally ill cancer patients, leading some authors to use the term "cancer anorexia-cachexia syndrome" (CACS) to describe this clinical condition.[7, 8]

Body weight loss has largely represented the cornerstone of cachexia diagnosis and staging. It can vary significantly according to cancer location and stage and is directly related to a worse clinical outcome and prognosis. However, body weight is influenced by a number of physiological and pathological changes (such as water retention, fat store replenishment, intracellular and extracellular water distribution alterations) and may in certain clinical conditions have low diagnostic accuracy. Therefore, although body weight loss was in the past the main diagnostic determinant, recent definition and classification has highlighted the preeminent role of body composition derangements in identifying cachectic patients.

Weight-losing patients suffered a loss of both fat and lean body mass. The loss of lean body mass, most notably skeletal muscle, is more dramatic in cancer patients and represents an independent predictor of morbidity and mortality.[9-13] A systematic literary review has revealed that there is a limited correlation between muscle mass and muscle function: muscle strength in lung cancer patients seemed to be affected regardless of loss of muscle mass. In patients with pre-cachexia, exercise capacity was significantly reduced, despite maintenance of muscle mass, and resistance exercise training increased all parameters of muscle strength and physical performance, with no difference to muscle mass.[9]

Low muscle mass associated with low muscle function (*i.e.* strength and performance) are features of the clinical condition called sarcopenia, which is a key diagnostic criterion for the definition of cancer cachexia, as mentioned above.[4] In various populations with cancer, sarcopenia is associated with poorer performance status (PS),[10] reduced overall survival [11] and an increased risk of chemotherapy toxicities.[12, 13]

Muscle degradation in the face of adequate nutrition is induced by both inflammatory cytokines and procachectic factors and is highly dependent on the patient's immune response. IL-6, TNF-α, and proteolysis inducing factor (PIF) are major contributors to the syndrome of muscle wasting in cancer patients.[14] The common pathway for muscle degradation involves ubiquitin-proteasome. Upstream activation is performed primarily through the NF-κB and STAT3 pathways, making them targets for potential interventions. Cytokines are important not only to establish tumor-host interaction and deregulate inflammatory response to tumor burden, but also as mediators of muscle wasting by directly targeting muscle tissue. In this regard, cachexia appears to be a genetically regulated response, dependent on a specific subset of genes, which control a highly regulated process of muscle protein degradation.[14] In clinical practice, several easily identifiable factors have been studied in an attempt to quantify the degree of inflammation and use that data to predict outcomes or guide treatment. The most commonly used inflammatory markers are represented by the elevated neutrophil: lymphocyte ratio (NLR), the C-reactive protein and the modified Glasgow Prognostic Score, which have been associated with impaired clinical outcomes.[15-17]

Inflammation and sarcopenia may be concurrently present in overweight/obese cancer patients: sarcopenic obesity appeared to be an additional prognostic risk factor [18] leading to lower pathological complete response rate and shorter progression-free survival to anticancer therapies.[19] In cancer patients affected by sarcopenic obesity, and the loss of lean body mass is notably related to poor survival, irrespective of age, sex, and functional status.[10] Thus, even in obese cancer patients, in which low-grade weight loss or stable body weight may be registered, the detection of body composition alterations and/or functional impairment should always be a guide to a more accurate assessment for the diagnosis of sarcopenia and/or cachexia that may significantly impair clinical outcome.

REFERENCES

1. Lucia S, Esposito M, Rossi Fanelli F, Muscaritoli M. Cancer cachexia: from molecular mechanisms to patient's care. Crit Rev Oncog 2012;17:315-21.
2. Muscaritoli M, Anker SD, Argiles J, Aversa Z, Bauer JM, Biolo G et al. Consensus definition of sarcopenia, cachexia and pre-cachexia: joint document elaborated by Special Interest Groups (SIG) "cachexia-anorexia in chronic wasting diseases" and "nutrition in geriatrics." Clin Nutr 2010;29:154-9.
3. Dewys WD, Begg C, Lavin PT, Band PR, Bennett JM, Bertino JR et al. Prognostic effect of weight loss prior to chemotherapy in cancer patients. Am J Med 1980;69:491-7.
4. Fearon K, Strasser F, Anker SD, Bosaeus I, Bruera E, Fainsinger RL et al. Definition and classification of cancer cachexia: an international consensus. Lancet Oncol 2011;12:489-95.
5. Muscaritoli M, Lucia S, Molfino A, Cederholm T, Rossi Fanelli F. Muscle atrophy in aging and chronic diseases: is it sarcopenia or cachexia? Intern Emerg Med 2013;8:553-60.
6. Vaughan VC, Martin P, Lewandowski PA. Cancer cachexia: impact, mechanisms and emerging treatments. J Cachexia Sarcopenia Muscle 2013;4:95-109.
7. Laviano A, Meguid MM, Inui A, Muscaritoli M, Rossi-Fanelli F. Therapy insight: Cancer anorexia-cachexia syndrome--when all you can eat is yourself. Nat Clin Pract Oncol 2005;2:158-65.
8. Muliawati Y, Haroen H, Rotty LW. Cancer anorexia - cachexia syndrome. Acta Med Indones 2012;44:154-62.
9. Collins J, Noble S, Chester J, Coles B, Byrne A. The assessment and impact of sarcopenia in lung cancer: a systematic literature review. BMJ Open 2014;4:e003697.
10. Prado CM, Lieffers JR, McCargar LJ, Reiman T, Sawyer MB, Martin L et al. Prevalence and clinical implications of sarcopenic obesity in patients with solid tumours of the respiratory and gastrointestinal tracts: a population-based study. Lancet Oncol 2008;9:629-35.
11. Harimoto N, Shirabe K, Yamashita YI, Ikegami T, Yoshizumi T, Soejima Y et al. Sarcopenia as a predictor of prognosis in patients following hepatectomy for hepatocellular carcinoma. Br J Surg 2013;100:1523-30.
12. Mir O, Coriat R, Blanchet B, Durand JP, Boudou-Rouquette P, Michels J et al. Sarcopenia predicts early dose-limiting toxicities and pharmacokinetics of sorafenib in patients with hepatocellular carcinoma. PLoS ONE 2012;7:e37563.
13. Prado CM, Baracos VE, McCargar LJ, Reiman T, Mourtzakis M, Tonkin K et al. Sarcopenia as a determinant of chemotherapy toxicity and time to tumor progression in metastatic breast cancer patients receiving capecitabine treatment. Clin Cancer Res 2009;15:2920-6.
14. Onesti JK, Guttridge DC. Inflammation based regulation of cancer cachexia. Biomed Res Int. 2014;2014:168407. Epub 2014 May 4.
15. Richards CH, Roxburgh CSD, MacMilla MR, Isswiasi S, Robertson EG, Guthrie GK et al. The relationships between body composition and the systemic inflammatory response in patients with primary operable colorectal cancer. PLoS ONE 2012;7:e41883.
16. Trutschnigg B, Kilgour RD, Morais JA, Lucar E, Hornby L, Molla H et al. Metabolic, nutritional and inflammatory characteristics in elderly women with advanced cancer. J Geriatr Oncol 2013;4:183-9.
17. Wu J, Huang C, Xiao H, Tang Q, Cai W. Weight loss and resting energy expenditure in male patients with newly diagnosed esophageal cancer. Nutrition 2013;29:1310-4.
18. Tan BH, Birdsell LA, Martin L, Baracos VE, Fearon KC. Sarcopenia in an overweight or obese patient is an adverse prognostic factor in pancreatic cancer. Clin Cancer Res 2009; 15:6973-9. Epub 2009 Nov 3.
19. Del Fabbro E, Parsons H, Warneke CL, Pulivarthi K, Litton JK, Dev R et al. The relationship between body composition and response to neoadjuvant chemotherapy in women with operable breast cancer. Oncologist 2012;17:1240-5. Epub 2012 Aug 17.

IMPACT OF CANCER CACHEXIA ON PATIENT OUTCOMES

S. LUCIA, M. MUSCARITOLI

INTRODUCTION

Cancer is a major public health problem across the world, particularly in western countries where it represents the second leading cause of death after heart disease, accounting for 23% of all deaths. It has been estimated that 13.7 million Americans with a history of cancer were alive on January 1, 2012 and that one in three women and one in two men in the United States will develop cancer in their lifetime.[1] Cancer survivors, defined as any person who has been diagnosed with cancer, are increasing, largely due to population aging, earlier diagnosis and improvement in treatments.[1] The increasing number of cancer survivors mean that current clinical practice must embrace new clinical issues, such as nutritional and metabolic support, in the attempt to improve patient outcomes. In parallel with the well-known increased prevalence of cancer diagnosis and cancer survivors,[2] the prevalence and the incidence of cancer cachexia is increasing[3] and the growing number of scientific works on this topic testify to the current direction of the scientific community's attention (e.g. when entering "cancer cachexia" on PubMed the result is noteworthy: 172 scientific works in 2011, 233 in 2012, 238 in 2013 and 197 to October 2014) (Fig. 2.1).

As seen in the previous chapter, cancer cachexia is phenotypically characterized by anorexia, weight loss, inflammation, body composition derangement and sarcopenia. All these features contribute alone or in combination to promote clinical deterioration and significantly impact patient outcomes.

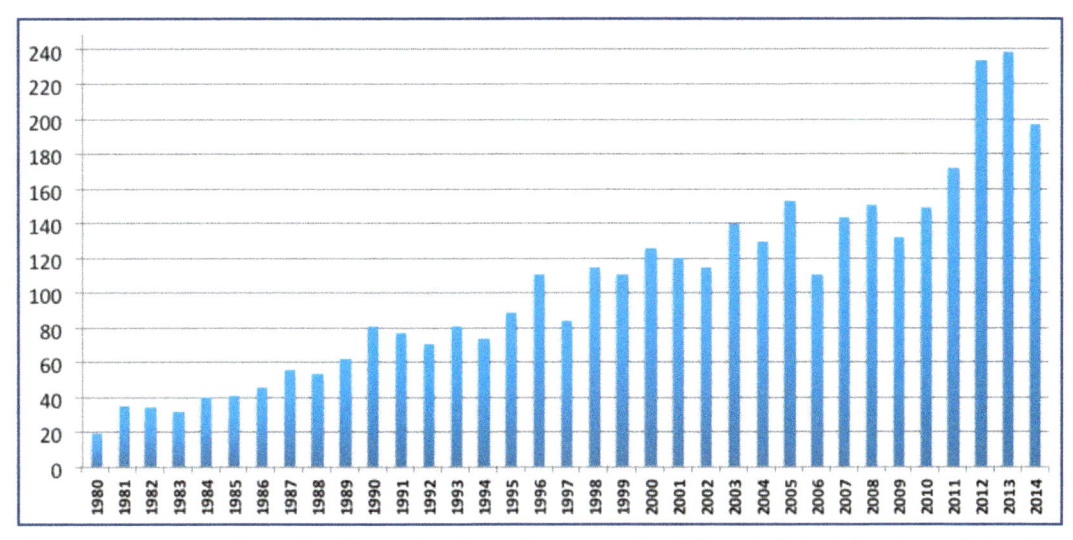

Figure 2.1 – Increasing scientific works about "cancer cachexia" on PubMed (yearly until October 2014).

Patient outcomes are interpreted here not only as a mere clinical endpoint but rather as the direct consequence of the results of interventions by the health care team, a concept involving the patient's well-being in a way more similar to the meaning of "prognosis". Clinical outcome is comprised of several aspects affecting cancer patients, such as survival, psychological distress, fatigue, pain, chronic inflammation, quality of life (QoL), physical activity, altered metabolism and body composition derangements (some of these are included in the cancer cachexia classification and are not therefore illustrated in this chapter). Morbidity and mortality, as comprehensive parameters to characterize patient outcomes, are the best prognostic indicators to describe the impact of cachexia on cancer patients.

PHYSICAL ACTIVITY AND PERFORMANCE STATUS (PS)

In patients affected by cancer cachexia, progressive impairment in physical function appears to be correlated with the loss of lean body mass, in particular skeletal muscle mass. Although the mechanisms implicated in muscle atrophy and sarcopenia are different (e.g. hyperactivation cytokine-dependent pathways, reduced protein anabolism and accelerated muscle catabolism), the final result of such modifications may lead to limited mobility and physical inactivity.[4-7]

Dahele et al. have demonstrated significant reductions in physical activity in advanced cancer patients receiving chemotherapy and have also indicated that patients with upper gastrointestinal cancer undergoing palliative chemotherapy had an overall reduction in median estimated total energy expenditure of about 8% when compared to age-matched healthy controls engaged in low-level recreational activity.[4] In cancer patients, physical activity was also correlated with both weight loss and BMI.[5] Since physical activity is impaired in cancer patients and is significantly related to a worse clinical outcome, physical exercise has been suggested as a promising intervention strategy for the prevention and treatment of cancer cachexia.[6] Aerobic and resistance physical exercise both promote physical activity by increasing lean body mass, muscle strength and function as well as by improving cardiovascular fitness.[5, 7]

Functional and performance status (PS) have been recognized as prognostic factors in several types of cancer and they represent a major independent prognostic factor for overall survival at all cancer stages, even in early localized disease.[8] The methods widely used for assessing the functional status of cancer patients are Karnofsky's index of performance status (KPS) and the Eastern Cooperative Oncology Group Performance Status Scale (ECOG PS).[9] Despite the method used, PS has been shown to be related to worse clinical outcomes and it is usually monitored during anticancer therapy in order to establish the efficacy of a specific intervention, since it has a highly predictive role in discriminating patients with bad prognosis.[10]

QUALITY OF LIFE

Quality of life (QoL) is supposed to describe how a person feels and how he or she functions. Although quality of life is certainly important in the broad sense, unfortunately, there is no unambiguous physical measurement or definable property which corresponds to "Quality of life". QoL is therefore measured using a brief questionnaire in which patients rate their ability to function in various ways and to enjoy life. Patients typically fill out the questionnaire several times during the course of a trial. The most commonly used questionnaire is the Functional Assessment of Cancer Therapy (FACT),[11] and there are specialized FACT questionnaires for several different types of cancer. QoL is a cornerstone of the modern comprehensive approach to cancer patients.[8, 12, 13] Beyond the feeling of well-being, QoL is strictly related to weight gain, physical strength and function, supporting the consistency of this outcome to predict clinical prognosis.[14] Decreased quality of life scores have been shown to be accompanied by significant decreases in physical activity and exercise capacity, which is strongly related to weight loss.[15] Cachexia negatively impacts surgical risk and responses to chemotherapy and radiotherapy, and ultimately results in decreased quality of life.[15] Cancer patients experiencing weight loss leading up to and during chemotherapy receive a lower initial dose and experience more frequent and severe dose-limiting toxicity when compared to weight-stable patients, consequently receiving significantly less treatment.[15] Assessing QoL can be onerous for patients and time-consuming for health professionals, as it often requires the completion of tools, sometimes complex and challenging, but it remains a valid clinical tool in both clinical care and research trials. QoL should be always assessed and monitored as it gives precious information for both prognosis and intervention efficacy. A recent systematic review highlighted the need for a specific instrument for cancer cachexia in order to properly detect emotional, social and cultural domains in such trials.[13]

PSYCHOLOGICAL DISTRESS

Although sometimes neglected, cancer and the various treatments employed to combat this disease have an impact on food intake that is psychological in nature. Intense psychological distress occurs in response to reduced appetite and food intake, increases in fatigue and significant alterations in appearance.[16] Symptoms such as food aversions, changes in food preferences and palatability, anticipatory nausea, vomiting and functional decline are sometimes interpreted by patients as a refractory condition with an inescapable destiny that produces emotional responses of anxiety and depression that in turn impact negatively on QoL, PS and survival.[15] There are also attitudinal responses, wherein social, religious, cultural, and other values related to food that may change as a consequence of the disease and may contribute to exacerbating psychological distress. Cancer patient families often rationalize that if food intake is increased, weight will be regained and survival increased, and that a failure to increase intake is equivalent to an incipient end.[17] This often leads to conflict between the patient and their family, as the patient's refusal of food is interpreted as a rejection of care and support, increasing anxieties over food and ultimately contributing to a decreased quality of life.[15] Although sometimes misleading and unrecognized, cachexia is a clinical condition that has profound psychological as well as physiological implications for patients and their families. In cancer patients, particularly when cachexia is present, more efforts should be focused on the early detection and treatment of psychological distress in order to increase QoL and PS and to make healthcare intervention more efficacious.

SURVIVAL

Survival is the best clinical outcome. It is generally the major goal of cancer treatment, although other outcomes (such as QoL and performance status) are also considered to better define clinical benefit. The first evidence of the impact of cancer cachexia on mortality was given by Dewys et al. in 1980, describing a shorter median survival rate and an increased treatment toxicity in cancer patients affected by cachexia-induced weight loss.[18] In the following years, lower survival rates was registered in several types of cancers and in different stages of disease (pancreatic cancer patients are illustrated in

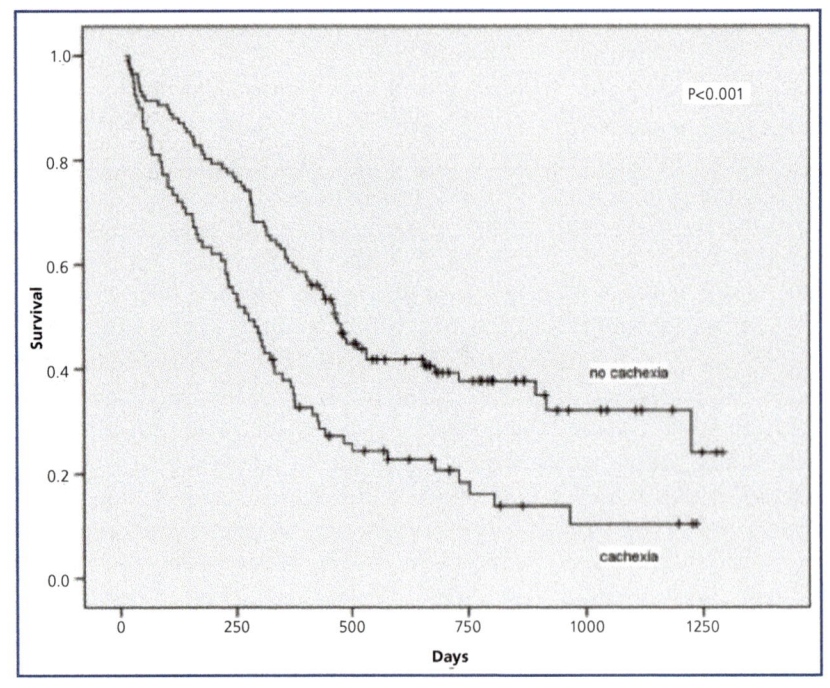

Figure 2.2 – Survival rates in pancreatic cancer patients showing significantly longer survival in patients without cachexia (P <0.001). Adapted from Bachmann et al.[21].

figure 2.2)[19-22] leading the attention of the scientific community to be focused on counteracting the main clinical determinants of cancer cachexia [22] in order to adequately and promptly treat this devastating condition.[1] Even in the early stages of renal cell carcinoma patients (T1N0M0), the presence of cachexia was associated with markedly worse disease-specific survival.[23] Cancer cachexia can affect survival, both facilitating clinical deterioration and reducing tolerance to anticancer therapies.[24] Additionally, oncologists significantly reduce or even stop chemotherapy or radiotherapy when cancer patients present cachexia-related signs, thus contributing to lower survival. Survival is correlated with a number of clinical and biochemical alterations that represent the main targets of cancer cachexia treatment, however, since cancer cachexia is a complex multi-factorial syndrome and no single agent has to date improved survival alone, the strategy of intervention must be multimodal and tailored to the patient's need in order to be effective.[1]

REFERENCES

1. Muscaritoli M, Molfino A, Lucia S, Rossi Fanelli F. Cachexia: A preventable comorbidity of cancer. A T.A.R.G.E.T. approach. Crit Rev Oncol Hematol. 2014 Nov 7. [Epub ahead of print].
2. DeSantis CE, Lin CC, Mariotto AB, Siegel RL, Stein KD, Kramer JL et al. Cancer treatment and survivorship statistics, 2014. CA Cancer J Clin 2014;64:252-71.
3. von Haehling S, Anker SD. Cachexia as a major underestimated and unmet medical need: facts and numbers. J Cachexia Sarcopenia Muscle 2010;1:1-5.
4. Dahele M, Skipworth RJ, Wall L, Voss A, Preston T, Fearon KC. Objective physical activity and self-reported quality of life in patients receiving palliative chemotherapy. J Pain Symptom Manage 2007;33:676-85.
5. Ravasco P, Monteiro-Grillo I, Vidal PM, Camilo ME. Cancer: disease and nutrition are key determinants of patients' quality of life. Support Care Cancer 2004;12:246-52.
6. Gould DW, Lahart I, Carmichael AR, Koutedakis Y, Metsios GS. Cancer cachexia prevention via physical exercise: molecular mechanisms. J Cachexia Sarcopenia Muscle 2013;4:111-24.

7. Stene GB, Helbostad JL, Balstad TR, Riphagen II, Kaasa S, Oldervoll LM. Effect of physical exercise on muscle mass and strength in cancer patients during treatment--a systematic review. Crit Rev Oncol Hematol 2013;88:573-93.
8. Tas F, Sen F, Odabas H, Kılıc L, Keskın S, Yıldız I. Performance status of patients is the major prognostic factor at all stages of pancreatic cancer. Int J Clin Oncol 2013;18:839-46.
9. Capuano G, Gentile PC, Bianciardi F, Tosti M, Palladino A, Di Palma M. Prevalence and influence of malnutrition on quality of life and performance status in patients with locally advanced head and neck cancer before treatment. Support Care Cancer 2010;18:433-7.
10. Buccheri G, Ferrigno D, Tamburini M. Karnofsky and ECOG performance status scoring in lung cancer: a prospective, longitudinal study of 536 patients from a single institution. Eur J Cancer 1996;32A:1135-41.
11. Cella DF, Tulsky DS, Gray G, Sarafian B, Linn E, Bonomi A et al. The Functional Assessment of Cancer Therapy scale: development and validation of the general measure. J Clin Oncol 1993;11:570-9.
12. Reck M, Thatcher N, Smit EF, Lorigan P, Szutowicz-Zielinska E, Liepa AM et al. Baseline quality of life and performance status as prognostic factors in patients with extensive-stage disease small cell lung cancer treated with pemetrexed plus carboplatin vs. etoposide plus carboplatin. Lung Cancer 2012;78:276-81.
13. Wheelwright S, Darlington AS, Hopkinson JB, Fitzsimmons D, White A, Johnson CD. A systematic review of health-related quality of life instruments in patients with cancer cachexia. Support Care Cancer 2013;21:2625-36.
14. Parmar MP, Swanson T, Jagoe RT. Weight changes correlate with alterations in subjective physical function in advanced cancer patients referred to a specialized nutrition and rehabilitation team. Support Care Cancer 2013;21:2049-57.
15. Vaughan VC, Martin P, Lewandowski A. Cancer cachexia: impact, mechanisms and emerging treatments. J Cachexia Sarcopenia Muscle 2013;4:95-109.
16. Strasser F, Binswanger J, Cerny T, Kesselring A. Fighting a losing battle: eating-related distress of men with advanced cancer and their female partners. A mixed-methods study. Palliat Med 2007;21:129-37.
17. Reid J, McKenna H, Fitzsimons D, McCance T. Fighting over food: patient and family understanding of cancer cachexia. Oncol Nurs Forum 2009;36:439-45.
18. Dewys WD, Begg C, Lavin PT, Band PR, Bennett JM, Bertino JR et al. Prognostic Effect of Weight Loss Prior to Chemotherapy in Cancer Patients. Am J Med 1980;69:491-7.
19. Kovarik M, Hronek M, Zadak Z. Clinically relevant determinants of body composition, function and nutritional status as mortality predictors in lung cancer patients. Lung Cancer 2014;84:1-6.
20. Couch M, Lai V, Cannon T, Guttridge D, Zanation A, George J et al. Cancer cachexia syndrome in head and neck cancer patients: part I. Diagnosis, impact on quality of life andsurvival, and treatment. Head Neck 2007;29:401-11.
21. Bachmann J, Ketterer K, Marsch C, Fechtner K, Krakowski-Roosen H, Büchler MW et al. Pancreatic cancer related cachexia: influence on metabolism and correlation to weight loss and pulmonary function. BMC Cancer 2009;9:255.
22. Blum D, Omlin A, Baracos VE, Solheim TS, Tan BH, Stone P et al.; European Palliative Care Research Collaborative. Cancer cachexia: a systematic literature review of items and domains associated with involuntary weight loss in cancer. Crit Rev Oncol Hematol 2011;80:114-44.
23. Kim HL, Han KR, Zisman A, Figlin RA, Belldegrun AS. Cachexia-like symptoms predict a worse prognosis in localized t1 renal cell carcinoma. J Urol 2004;171:1810-3.
24. Fearon K, Strasser F, Anker SD, Bosaeus I, Bruera E, Fainsinger RL et al. Definition and classification of cancer cachexia: an international consensus. Lancet Oncol 2011;12:489-95.

BIOCHEMICAL FEATURES OF MUSCLE WASTING IN CANCER CACHEXIA

P. COSTELLI, Z. AVERSA

INTRODUCTION

Muscle wasting is by far the most clinically relevant feature of cancer cachexia and reflects increased protein degradation, reduced protein synthesis or a relative imbalance of the two.[1] One of the consequences of muscle wasting is the increase in peripheral release of aminoacids, which can be utilized by various tissues and organs, such as the liver for acute phase proteins synthesis and gluconeogenesis.[2] The accelerated loss of muscle mass with disease progression has a negative impact on patient morbidity and mortality, quality of life and response to anti-neoplastic treatments.[3] Moreover, the progressive loss of muscle mass is associated with a reduction in muscle strength and function that may result in reduced physical activity which in turn can further exacerbate muscle loss thus creating a vicious cycle.

The precise mechanisms that mediate muscle loss are not completely understood, but different molecular pathways have been involved. Studies performed on experimental models of cancer cachexia as well as in cancer patients have shown that increased protein degradation plays a predominant role, although alteration in muscle protein synthesis may contribute as well.[4]

A complex interplay among cytokines, hormones and other humoral factors is involved in the upstream derangement of muscle trophism typical of cancer cachexia.[5] In addition alterations in energy and substrate metabolism, reduction in nutrient intake and/or availability (secondary to anorexia, malabsorption, and anti-neoplastic treatments) and reduced mobility may contribute as well to the pathogenesis of cancer cachexia.[6]

This chapter will focus on the main molecular mechanisms which have been implicated in the pathogenesis of muscle wasting in cancer cachexia (Fig. 3.1).

CATABOLIC RESPONSE

The enhanced muscle protein breakdown in cancer cachexia relies on the activity of different degradative mechanisms such as the ubiquitin-proteasome system, the authophagic-lysosomal pathway and the calcium-dependent proteases (calpains).

In the ubiquitin-proteasome system, proteins are targeted for degradation by the 26S proteasome complex through the ATP-dependent addition of a ubiquitin chain. The 26S proteolytic complex consists of one or two 19S regulatory particles and the core 20S proteasome which is characterized by five peptidase activities: trypsin-like, chimotrypsin-like, peptidyl-glutamyl peptidase, branched-chain amino acid-preferring and small-neutral amino acid-preferring activities. The ubiquitin chain is attached to the protein substrate through an enzymatic cascade involving the ubiquitin activating enzymes (E1), the ubiquitin conjugating enzymes (E2) and the ubiquitin ligases (E3); these latters bind the protein substrates and catalyze the transfer of the ubiquitin from the E2 enzymes to the substrate.[7] This is a rate-limiting step as once the protein is ubiquitylated it is docked to the proteasome for degradation

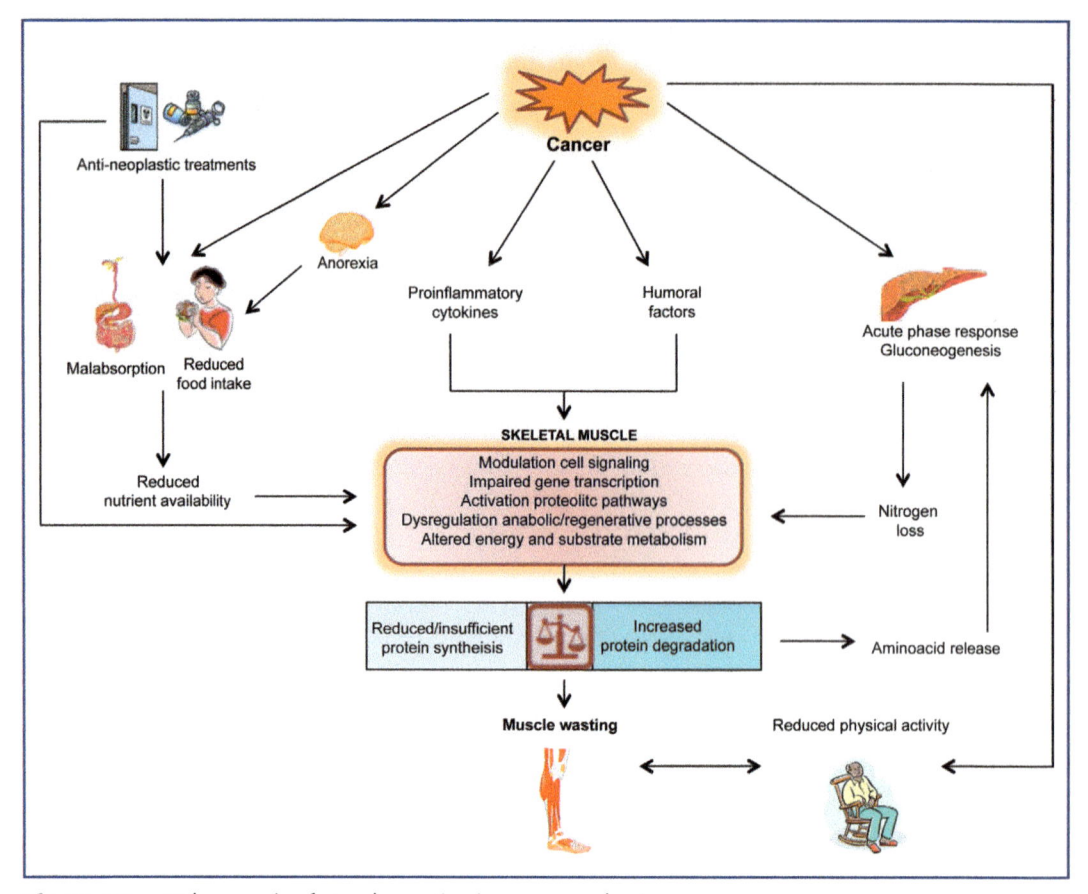

Figure 3.1 – Pathogenesis of muscle wasting in cancer cachexia.

unless the polyubiquitin chain is removed by the de-ubiquitinating enzymes.[8] Several E3s have been described, but only a few have been found to regulate muscle atrophy, such as atrogin-1/MAFbx and MuRF1.[9, 10] Knockout mice for either MuRF1 or atrogin-1/MAFbx were shown to be resistant to muscle atrophy [10] and increased atrogin-1/MAFbx and MuRF1 mRNA levels were reported in experimental models of cancer cachexia.[11-13]

Activation of the ubiquitin-proteasome pathway has been observed in the skeletal muscle of tumor-bearing animals [14, 15] as well as in patients with pancreatic, gastric and liver cancer.[16-19] Interestingly, both ubiquitin mRNA overexpression and increased proteasome proteolytic activities have been reported in gastric cancer patients even with insignificant or no weight loss, supporting the concept that the causative mechanisms of cancer cachexia are operating early during the clinical course of neoplastic disease.[18] Other studies, however, have reported no changes in the ubiquitin-proteasome system activity in muscle biopsies from non-small cell lung cancer patients with weight loss <10% [20] and esophageal cancer patients [21], suggesting that differences in the ubiquitin-proteasome pathway involvement in muscle wasting may exist among different tumour types.

Besides the ubiquitin-proteasome system, autophagy is another important contributor to muscle wasting. Autophagy is a highly conserved homeostatic mechanism for degradation of cellular constituents that increases under stress conditions leading to organelle damage or under marked nutrient restriction to recycle biomolecules for the synthesis of essential constituents.[22] Three different types of autophagy have been described: macroautophagy, microautophagy, and chaperone-mediated autophagy.[23] Macroautophagy is considered the major type of autophagy and recent findings suggest that it plays a central role in the regulation of muscle mass.[8] In macroautophagy, a portion of cytoplasm, including organelles, is engulfed by an isolation membrane (phagophore) to form an autophagosome. The autophagosome fuses with the lysosome forming an autolysosome where the autophagosome cargo is degraded.[24] Although autophagy was initially considered a non-selective degradation pathway, it is now becoming increasingly evident that it can trigger the selective removal of protein aggregates or specific organelles such as mitochondria via mithophagy or ribosomes via ribophagy.[8,25] The selectivity of autophagic degradation is conferred by specific cargo signals such as p62, Bnip3, Nbr1, which have both a cargo-binding domain (that recognizes and attaches organelles) and a LC3-interaction domain, that recruits and binds essential autophagosome membrane proteins. Adaptor proteins are able to recognize their target by specific flag molecules or post-translational modifications, such as ubiquitination, presented on the surface of the cargo.[26]

Increased autophagy flux has been reported in several conditions characterized by modulations of muscle mass, such as fasting or exercise.[27-29] Conversely, an impairment of autophagy with accumulation of unfolded and aggregate-prone proteins and dysfunctional organelles is a typical feature of several myopathies.[30,31] Disorders in which autophagic vacuoles are seen in the skeletal muscle are generally referred to as authophagic vacuolar myopathies which include Pompe disease and Danon disease.[32] Recently, defective autophagy has been demontrated to contribute also to the pathogenesis of different forms of muscular dystrophies which could display either accumulation of altered organelles inside myofibers (impaired autophagy), or excessive degradation of myofiber components (excess autophagy).[8]

Autophagy is induced in the skeletal muscle also in different catabolic conditions including cancer. Recently, indeed, autophagy has been shown to contribute to muscle atrophy in three different experimental models of cancer cachexia.[33] In addition a modulation of the autophagic-lysosomal pathway has been observed in the skeletal muscle of esophageal cancer patients[21] as well as in lung cancer patients.[34]

Finally, the calcium-dependent proteolysis relies on the activity of calpains, a family of calcium-dependent cysteine-proteases whose regulation is complex and not completely elucidated. Calpains may play a critical role in initiating the breakdown of myofibrillar proteins by releasing substrates suitable for further degradation by the proteasome system. Increased m-calpain and reduced p94 calpain (a negative regulator of calcium-dependent proteolysis) expression have been found in rats bearing the AH-130 ascites hepatoma.[35,36] In addition, increased calpain activity measured in vitro as well as reduction of two calpain substrates (calpastatin and the 130kDa calcium-ATPase) have been reported in the same experimental model.[37] Interestingly, calpain activity has been found increased in the skeletal muscle of gastric cancer patients with minimal or no-weight loss suggesting that activation of the calcium-dependent proteolysis in the skeletal muscle may be an early response to cancer.[38] By contrast, no change in calpain activity has been observed in esophageal cancer patients suggesting that differences among tumor types could occur.[21]

In addition to the degradative systems described above, there are some evidences indicating that apoptosis may play a role as well in the pathogenesis of cancer-related muscle wasting. An increase in the activity of caspases, the enzymes associated with the execution of apoptosis, was observed in the gastrocnemius of MAC16 bearing mice [39] and DNA fragmentation typical of apoptosis was found in the skeletal muscle of Yoshida AH-130 ascites hepatoma-bearing rats and Lewis Lung carcinoma-bearing mice.[40] Despite these observations in experimental models, an initial study found no evidence for increased apoptosis in the *rectus abdominis* of gastric cancer patients,[41] whereas a following study on muscle biopsies from weight losing upper gastrointestinal cancer patients showed a significant increase in DNA fragmentation and in poly (adenosine diphosphate-ribose) polymerase (PARP) cleavage indicating the presence of apoptosis.[42] However, recently no change in caspase-3 activity was found in muscle biopsies from esophageal cancer patients.[21] The reason for such discrepancies is not known but may be related to differences in both tumour types and staging, as well as differences in the rate of muscle atrophy.

ANABOLIC RESPONSE

Although muscle protein degradation plays a major role in the pathogenesis of muscle wasting in cancer cachexia, perturbations in the anabolic signaling may occur as well. One of the best characterized anabolic pathways in the regulation of muscle mass is the insulin-like growth factor-1 (IGF-1)-dependent signaling. IGF-1 is an anabolic growth factor that stimulates muscle protein synthesis as well as proliferation and differentiation of satellite cells.[43] It exerts antiapoptotic effects on muscle cells, suppresses proteolysis and inhibits the ubiquitin-proteasome system.[15, 44] The effects exerted by IGF-1 on muscles mainly result from stimulation of the phosphatidylinositol-3 kinase (PI3K)/Akt pathway, leading to activation of downstream targets required for protein synthesis by blocking repression of the mammalian target of rapamycin (mTOR).[45] Interestingly, this kinase plays an important role also in the regulation of the autophagyc-lysosomal degradation: indeed nutrients, especially free amino acids, are sensed by the mTOR kinase which inhibits autophagy by blocking the formation of the Atg/ULK complex, an important regulatory step for autophagy initiation.[8] In addition, mTOR inhibits the transcription factor EB (TFEB) which is a master regulator of lysosome biogenesis.[46]

In the last years several reports have proposed that signaling through the PI3K/Akt pathway also inhibits the expression of the muscle-specific ubiquitin ligases atrogin-1 and MuRF1 by inactivating the Forkhead box class O (FoxO) transcription factors.[47, 48] Accordingly, FoxO-1 silencing has been shown to prevent protein degradation in a murine model of cancer cachexia.[49] Interestingly, besides promoting atrogin-1 and MuRF1 gene transcription, FoxOs factors control other pathways involved in the regulation of muscle mass. Indeed, FoxO3 has been involved in the upregulation of autophagy-related genes as well as in the reduction of protein synthesis in atrophying muscles. These observations suggest that both Akt and FoxOs play an important role in the crosstalk between protein synthesis and degradation pathways, also by coordinating the activation of both the ubiquitin-proteasome system and autophagy during muscle wasting.[50, 51]

Perturbations of the IGF-1 signaling have been reported in both *in vivo* and *in vitro* models of muscle atrophy as well as in pathological conditions associated with muscle loss.[52-56] Results obtained in rats bearing the AH-130 tumor have shown reduced IGF-1 expression in both liver and skeletal muscle and recently decreased IGF-1 mRNA levels were detected also in muscle biopsies from gastric cancer patients with or without body weight loss.[11, 57] However, the anabolic pathway downstream to IGF-1 is not down-regulated in tumor-bearing animals, indicating that a compensatory mechanism to reduced IGF-1 and increased protein degradation may have occurred.[58] This pattern of IGF-1 activation differs from that reported in other experimental models of cancer cachexia [59,60] and in patients with pancreatic cancer.[61] Such discrepancy may be due either to different experimental and working conditions as well as to modulations of the IGF-1 axis peculiar to different tumor types.

Defective skeletal muscle regeneration may also contribute to muscle wasting in cancer cachexia. Recently both the expression of myogenic factors [58,62] and myogenic differentiation have been shown to be impaired in cancer hosts, contributing to muscle depletion.[58,63]

MEDIATORS OF MUSCLE WASTING

Several pro-inflammatory cytokines, including tumor necrosis factor-α (TNF-α), interleukin-1 (IL-1), interleukin-6 (IL-6) and interferon-γ (IFN-γ) have been postulated to play a role in the pathogenesis of cancer-related muscle wasting. Cytokines production during cancer cachexia is thought to derive from either the tumor or the host.[64] The effects of pro-inflammatory cytokines on muscle mass, particularly TNF-α, are at least in part mediated by the transcription factor NF-kB. Studies on experimental models suggest that NF-kB signaling is activated in the skeletal muscle during cancer cachexia [63,65] and recently a modulation of this transcription factor has been observed in gastric and lung cancer patients.[34,66]

TNF-α has been shown to induce cachexia in animal studies and to promote atrophy in cultured myotubes.[67,68] Besides inducing E3 ligase genes via NF-kB [68-70], TNF-α can cause insulin resistance [71] and, in combination with IFN-γ, it down-regulates, in a NF-kB dependent fashion, MyoD, a muscle specific transcription factor.[72] Although several evidences point to TNF-α as involved in experimental cancer cachexia, its role in human pathology remains questionable. Recent trials using TNF-α antibodies in cancer patients did not show any benefit [73] raising the possibility that TNF-α is a facilitator, but it is not sufficient to promote muscle wasting, and that the synergistic or additional activities of other tumor or host-derived factors are needed. Alternatively, the possibility that TNF-α mediates cachexia only in a subset of patients and that effective therapy would be possible only in this group of patients should be taken into account.[5]

Another wasting-associated cytokine is IL-6. Its serum levels are frequently elevated in tumor-bearing animals.[74] In addition, circulating levels of IL-6 correlate with weight loss in patients with advanced small cell lung cancer and colon cancer and influence survival in a variety of cancer types.[75-77] IL-6-dependent signaling relies on activation of the Janus kinase/signal transducers and activators of transcription (JAK/STAT) pathway.[78] Consistently, pharmacological or genetic inhibition of the JAK/STAT3 pathways in an experimental model of cancer cachexia has been reported to reduce muscle atrophy, suggesting that STAT3 is a causative factor as well as a therapeutic potential therapeutic target of muscle wasting.[79] Recent clinical trials have also tested a monoclonal anti-IL-6 antibody on lung cancer patients showing a reversal of anorexia, anemia and fatigue, but no effect on lean body mass.[80]

Much attention has been put on myostatin, a transforming growth factor-β (TGF-β) family member, also known as growth and differentiation factor-8 (GDF-8) that negatively regulates muscle mass.[81] Active myostatin binds the activin type II B receptor (ActRIIB) resulting in phosphorylation and activation of the transcription factors SMAD2 and 3 [mammalian homologue of Drosophila

MAD (Mothers-Against-Decapentaplegic gene)], which bind to SMAD4 and translocate into the nucleus regulating the expression of target genes.[82] Myostatin has also been suggested to exert its action through different pathways, such as the extracellular signal-regulated kinase (ERK)/ mitogen activated protein kinase (MAPK) cascade [83] and the Akt-FoxO1 signaling.[84]

Myostatin signaling is enhanced in the skeletal muscle of tumor-bearing rats and mice and myostatin inhibition, either by antisense oligonucleotides or by administration of an activin receptor II B/fragment-crystallizable (ActRIIB/Fc) fusion protein or ActRIIB-soluble form, prevent muscle wasting in tumor-bearing mice.[85, 86] Recent results obtained on muscle biopsies suggest that myostatin signaling is altered also in non weight-losing cancer patients, although different patterns of molecular changes may exist among different tumor types.[87]

ALTERED ENERGY AND SUBSTRATE METABOLISM

Increased resting energy expenditure (REE), most likely secondary to the imbalance between pro-inflammatory (TNF-α, IL-1, IL-6, IFN-γ) and anti-inflammatory (IL-4, IL-12, IL-15) cytokines, has been long considered an essential factor in the pathogenesis of cancer cachexia.[64] However, this view has been reconsidered based on the observation that the metabolic response to cancer may be extremely heterogeneous, some patients showing hypermetabolism, others being frankly hypometabolic.[88, 89] Indeed, in patients with overt cachexia and asthenia in spite of increased REE, total energy expenditure may be reduced as a consequence of decreased physical activity.[90]

Increased glycogenolysis and gluconeogenesis from amino acids and lactate (produced in excess by many tumors as a consequence of increased glucose uptake/glycolis), insulin resistance, enhanced protein turnover, increased fat oxidation and reduced lipogenesis are the prominent disturbances in energy substrate metabolism.[91]

Alterations of energy metabolism in muscle wasting conditions are suggested also by the occurrence of mitochondria abnormalities. These organelles play an important role in the control of skeletal muscle homeostasis as they provide most of the ATP required for metabolic cell processes via oxidative phosphorylation and adapt their morphology to the bioenergetic cell requirements by fusion and fission events.[92] Consistently, in IL-6-dependent cancer cachexia both oxidative capacity and mitochondria dynamics are reduced in oxidative and glycolytic muscles with severe wasting,[93] and mitochondrial dysfunction has been observed in the skeletal muscle of rats bearing the AH-130 hepatoma.[94]

The transcriptional cofactor perixosome proliferator-activated receptor γ coactivator 1α (PGC-1α) is a critical regulator of muscle oxidative capacity and mitochondrial biogenesis, and it is considered a key sensor of muscular activity. Indeed, muscle contraction results in mild oxidative stress, elevated AMP/ATP ratio and transient rise in cytoplasmic calcium concentration which activate various downstream pathways, such as p38-MAPK, the energy sensor AMP-activated protein kinase (AMPK) and the calcium-sensitive signaling, that can modulate the activity and expression of PGC-1α.[26, 92, 95] Besides being crucial in the maintenance of energy homeostasis, PGC-1α can also reduce protein breakdown by inhibiting the transcriptional activity of FoxO3 and NF-kB, without affecting protein synthesis.[96] Interestingly, reduced PGC-1α mRNA expression has been observed in the gastrocnemius muscles of tumor-bearing animals.[97] However, PGC-1α overexpression in the skeletal muscle of transgenic MCK-PGC-1α mice implanted with Lewis Lung carcinoma not only did not prevent muscle loss, but resulted in increased tumor growth.[98] In this regard, despite PGC-1α hyperexpressing skeletal muscle shows a switch to oxidative metabolism, increased mitochondrial content and improvements in physical endurance exercise, tissue mass is not particularly affected, suggesting that increased mitochondrial biogenesis per se does not lead to muscle hypertrophy.[92]

An important role in cell energy homeostasis is also played by AMPK, that besides regulating PGC-1α, is able to increase catabolism and decrease anabolism in response to reduced energy. Indeed, activated AMPK inhibits mTOR, activates Ulk1 and triggers FoxO3 to promote protein breakdown via autophagy and ubiquitin-proteasome pathway, thus producing alternative energy substrates and restoring ATP level.[92, 99] Interestingly, muscle AMPK activity is increased in Apc$^{min/+}$ mice engineered to hyperexpress IL-6 in the skeletal muscle.[100]

CONCLUSIONS

In conclusion, available experimental and clinical evidences show that muscle wasting in cancer cachexia results from profound metabolic alterations due to the combined action of factors released either by the tumor or by the host as well as to the effects of reduced nutrients availability, anti-neoplastic treatments and physical inactivity. This complex interplay among multiple signaling pathways is involved in altering the physiological balance between protein synthesis and breakdown rates eventually leading to the onset of a protein hypercatabolic state.

The growing amount of knowledge about the biochemical and molecular mechanisms underlying muscle wasting in cancer cachexia appears highly relevant to allow the development of future effective therapeutic interventions acting selectively at the muscle level.

REFERENCES

1. Glass DJ. Signaling pathways perturbing muscle mass. Curr Opin Clin Nutr Metab Care 2010; 13:225-9.
2. Vary TC, Kimball SR. Regulation of hepatic protein synthesis in chronic inflammation and sepsis. Am J Physiol 1992;262(2 Pt 1):C445-52.
3. Muscaritoli M, Molfino A, Gioia G, Laviano A, Rossi Fanelli F. The "parallel pathway": a novel nutritional and metabolic approach to cancer patients. Intern Emerg Med 2011;6:105-12.
4. Muscaritoli M, Bossola M, Aversa Z, Bellantone R, Rossi Fanelli F. Prevention and treatment of cancer cachexia: new insight into an old problem. Eur J Cancer 2006;42:31-41.
5. Fearon KC, Glass DJ, Guttridge DC. Cancer cachexia: mediators, signaling, and metabolic pathways. Cell Metab Rev 2012;16:153-66.
6. Muscaritoli M, Lucia S, Molfino A, Cederholm T, Rossi Fanelli F. Muscle atrophy in aging and chronic diseases: is it sarcopenia or cachexia? Intern Emerg Med 2013;8:553-60.
7. Ciechanover A. The ubiquitin-proteasome proteolytic pathway. Cell 1994;79:13-21.
8. Sandri M. Protein breakdown in muscle wasting: role of autophagy-lysosome and ubiquitine proteasome. Int J Biochem Cell Biol 2013;45:2121-9.
9. Gomes MD, Lecker SH, Jagoe RT, Navon A, Goldberg AL. Atrogin-1, a muscle-specific F-box protein highly expressed during muscle atrophy. Proc Natl Acad Sci USA 2001;98:14440-5.
10. Bodine SC, Latres E, Baumhueter S, Lai VK, Nunez L, Clarke BA et al. Identification of ubiquitin ligases required for skeletal muscle atrophy. Science 2001;294:1704-8.
11. Costelli P, Muscaritoli M, Bossola M, Penna F, Reffo P, Bonetto A et al. IGF-1 is downregulated in experimental cancer cachexia. J Physiol Regul Integr Comp Physiol 2006;291:R674-83.
12. Siddiqui RA, Hassan S, Harvey KA, Rasool T, Das T, Mukerji P et al. Attenuation of proteolysis and muscle wasting by curcumin c3 complex in MAC16 colon tumour-bearing mice. Br J Nutr 2009;102:967-75.
13. Penna F, Bonetto A, Muscaritoli M, Costamagna D, Minero VG, Bonelli G et al. Muscle atrophy in experimental cancer cachexia: is the IGF-1 signaling pathway involved? Int J Cancer 2010;127:1706-17.

14. Baracos VE, DeVivo C, Hoyle DH, Goldberg AL. Activation of the ATP-ubiquitin-proteasome pathway in skeletal muscle of cachectic rats bearing a hepatoma. Am J Physiol 1995; 268(5 Pt 1):E996-1006.
15. Lecker SH, Jagoe RT, Gilbert A, Gomes M, Baracos V, Bailey J et al. Multiple types of skeletal muscle atrophy involve a common program of changes in gene expression. FASEB J 2004;18:39-51.
16. Williams A, Sun X, Fischer JE, Hasselgren PO. The expression of genes in the ubiquitin-proteasome proteolytic pathway is increased in skeletal muscle from patients with cancer. Surgery 1999;126:744-9.
17. Bossola M, Muscaritoli M, Costelli P, Bellantone R, Pacelli F, Busquets S et al. Increased muscle ubiquitin mRNA levels in gastric cancer patients. Am J Physiol Regul Integr Comp Physiol 2001;280:R1518-23.
18. Bossola M, Muscaritoli M, Costelli P, Grieco G, Bonelli G, Pacelli F et al. Increased muscle proteasome activity correlates with disease severity in gastric cancer patients. Ann Surg 2003;237:384-9.
19. Khal J, Hine AV, Fearon KC, Dejong CH, Tisdale MJ. Increased expression of proteasome subunits in skeletal muscle of cancer patients with weight loss. Int J Biochem Cell Biol 2005;37:2196-206.
20. Op den Kamp CM, Langen RC, Minnaard R, Kelders MC, Snepvangers FJ, Hesselink MK et al. Pre-cachexia in patients with stages I-III non-small cell lung cancer: systemic inflammation and functional impairment without activation of skeletal muscle ubiquitin proteasome system. Lung Cancer 2012;76:112-7.
21. Tardif N, Klaude M, Lundell L, Thorell A, Rooyackers O. Autophagic-lysosomal pathway is the main proteolytic system modified in the skeletal muscle of esophageal cancer patients. Am J Clin Nutr 2013;98:1485-92.
22. Petiot A, Pattingre S, Arico S, Meley D, Codogno P. Diversity of signaling controls of macroautophagy in mammalian cells. Cell Struct Funct 2002; 27:431-41.
23. Mizushima N, Levine B, Cuervo AM, Klionsky DJ. Autophagy fights disease through cellular self-digestion. Nature 2008;451:1069-75.
24. Mizushima N, Komatsu M. Autophagy: renovation of cells and tissues. Cell 2011;147:728-41.
25. Singh R, Cuervo AM. Autophagy in the cellular energetic balance. Cell Metab 2011;13:495-504.
26. Vainshtein A, Grumati P, Sandri M, Bonaldo P. Skeletal muscle, autophagy, and physical activity: the ménage à trois of metabolic regulation in health and disease. J Mol Med (Berl) 2013 Nov 24. [Epub ahead of print].
27. Mammucari C, Milan G, Romanello V, Masiero E, Rudolf R, Del Piccolo P et al. FoxO3 controls autophagy in skeletal muscle in vivo. Cell Metab 2007;6:458-71.
28. O'Leary MF, Vainshtein A, Carter HN, Zhang Y, Hood DA. Denervation-induced mitochondrial dysfunction and autophagy in skeletal muscle of apoptosis-deficient animals. Am J Physiol Cell Physiol 2012;303:C447-54.
29. Grumati P, Coletto L, Schiavinato A, Castagnaro S, Bertaggia E, Sandri M et al. Physical exercise stimulates autophagy in normal skeletal muscles but is detrimental for collagen VI-deficient muscles. Autophagy 2011;7:1415-23.
30. Grumati P, Coletto L, Sabatelli P, Cescon M, Angelin A, Bertaggia E et al. Autophagy is defective in collagen VI muscular dystrophies, and its reactivation rescues myofiber degeneration. Nat Med 2010;16:1313-20.
31. Nogalska A, D'Agostino C, Terracciano C, Engel WK, Askanas V. Impaired autophagy in sporadic inclusion-body myositis and in endoplasmic reticulum stress-provoked cultured human muscle fibers. Am J Pathol 2010; 177:1377-87.
32. Malicdan MC, Nishino I. Autophagy in lysosomal myopathies. Brain Pathol 2012;22:82-8.
33. Penna F, Costamagna D, Pin F, Camperi A, Fanzani A, Chiarpotto EM et al. Autophagic degradation contributes to muscle wasting in cancer cachexia. Am J Pathol 2013;182:1367-78.
34. Op den Kamp CM, Langen RC, Snepvangers FJ, de Theije CC, Schellekens JM, Laugs F et al. Nuclear transcription factor κ B activation and protein turnover adaptations in skeletal muscle of patients with progressive stages of lung cancer cachexia. Am J Clin Nutr 2013;98:738-48.
35. Temparis S, Asensi M, Taillandier D, Aurousseau E, Larbaud D, Obled A et al. Increased ATP-ubiquitin-dependent proteolysis in skeletal muscles of tumor-bearing rats. Cancer Res 1994;54:5568-73.
36. Busquets S, García-Martínez C, Alvarez B, Carbó N, López-Soriano FJ, Argilés JM. Calpain-3 gene expression is decreased during ex-

perimental cancer cachexia. Biochim Biophys Acta 2000;1475:5-9.
37. Costelli P, Reffo P, Penna F, Autelli R, Bonelli G, Baccino FM. Ca (2+)-dependent proteolysis in muscle wasting. Int J Biochem Cell Biol 2005;37:2134-46.
38. Smith IJ, Aversa Z, Hasselgren PO, Pacelli F, Rosa F, Doglietto GB et al. Calpain activity is increased in skeletal muscle from gastric cancer patients with no or minimal weight loss. Muscle Nerve 2011;43:410-4.
39. Belizário JE, Lorite MJ, Tisdale MJ. Cleavage of caspases-1, -3, -6, -8 and -9 substrates by proteases in skeletal muscles from mice undergoing cancer cachexia. Br J Cancer 2001; 84:1135-40.
40. van Royen M, Carbó N, Busquets S, Alvarez B, Quinn LS, López-Soriano FJ et al. DNA fragmentation occurs in skeletal muscle during tumor growth: A link with cancer cachexia? Biochem Biophys Res Commun 2000; 270:533-7.
41. Bossola M, Mirabella M, Ricci E, Costelli P, Pacelli F, Tortorelli AP et al. Skeletal muscle apoptosis is not increased in gastric cancer patients with mild-moderate weight loss. Int J Biochem Cell Biol 2006;38:1561-70.
42. Busquets S, Deans C, Figueras M, Moore-Carrasco R, López-Soriano FJ, Fearon KC et al. Apoptosis is present in skeletal muscle of cachectic gastro-intestinal cancer patients. Clin Nutr 2007;26:614-8.
43. Florini JR, Ewton DZ, Coolican SA. Growth hormone and the insulin-like growth factor system in myogenesis. Endocr Rev 1996; 17:481-517.
44. Chrysis D, Underwood LE. Regulation of components of the ubiquitin system by insulin-like growth factor I and growth hormone in skeletal muscle of rats made catabolic with dexamethasone. Endocrinology 1999;140:5635-41.
45. Rommel C, Bodine SC, Clarke BA, Rossman R, Nunez L, Stitt TN et al. Mediation of IGF-1-induced skeletal myotube hypertrophy by PI(3)K/Akt/mTOR and PI(3)K/Akt/GSK3 pathways. Nat Cell Biol 2001;3:1009-13.
46. Settembre C, Di Malta C, Polito VA, Garcia Arencibia M, Vetrini F, Erdin S et al. TFEB links autophagy to lysosomal biogenesis. Science 2011; 332:1429-33.
47. Sandri M, Sandri C, Gilbert A, Skurk C, Calabria E, Picard A et al. Foxo transcription factors induce the atrophy-related ubiquitin ligase atrogin-1 and cause skeletal muscle atrophy. Cell 2004;117:399-412.
48. Stitt TN, Drujan D, Clarke BA, Panaro F, Timofeyva Y, Kline WO et al. The IGF-1/PI3K/Akt pathway prevents expression of muscle atrophy-induced ubiquitin ligases by inhibiting FOXO transcription factors. Mol Cell 2004;14:395-403.
49. Liu CM, Yang Z, Liu CW, Wang R, Tien P, Dale R et al. Effect of RNA oligonucleotide targeting Foxo-1 on muscle growth in normal and cancer cachexia mice. Cancer Gene Ther 2007;14:945-52.
50. Sandri M. Autophagy in skeletal muscle. FEBS Lett 2010;584:1411-6.
51. Bonaldo P, Sandri M. Cellular and molecular mechanisms of muscle atrophy. Dis Model Mech 2013;6:25-39.
52. Fan J, Molina PE, Gelato MC, Lang CH. Differential tissue regulation of insulin-like growth factor-I content and binding proteins after endotoxin. Endocrinology 1994; 134:1685-92.
53. Attard-Montalto SP, Camacho-Hübner C, Cotterill AM, D'Souza-Li L, Daley S, Bartlett K et al. Changes in protein turnover, IGF-I and IGF binding proteins in children with cancer. Acta Paediatr 1998;87:54-60.
54. Heszele MF, Price SR. Insulin-like growth factor I: the yin and yang of muscle atrophy. Endocrinology 2004;145:4803-5.
55. Sugiura T, Abe N, Nagano M, Goto K, Sakuma K, Naito H et al. Changes in PKB/Akt and calcineurin signaling during recovery in atrophied soleus muscle induced by unloading. Am J Physiol Regul Integr Comp Physiol 2005;288:R1273-8.
56. Schakman O, Kalista S, Bertrand L, Lause P, Verniers J, Ketelslegers JM et al. Role of Akt/GSK-3beta/beta-catenin transduction pathway in the muscle anti-atrophy action of insulin-like growth factor-I in glucocorticoid-treated rats. Endocrinology 2008;149:3900-8.
57. Bonetto A, Penna F, Aversa Z, Mercantini P, Baccino FM, Costelli P et al. Early changes of muscle insulin-like growth factor-1 and myostatin gene expression in gastric cancer patients. Muscle Nerve 2013;48:387-92.
58. Penna F, Costamagna D, Fanzani A, Bonelli G, Baccino FM, Costelli P. Muscle wasting

and impaired myogenesis in tumor bearing mice are prevented by ERK inhibition. PLoS One 2010;5:e13604.
59. Eley HL, Russell ST, Tisdale MJ. Effect of branched-chain amino acids on muscle atrophy in cancer cachexia. Biochem J 2007; 407:113-20.
60. Asp ML, Tian M, Wendel AA, Belury MA. Evidence for the contribution of insulin resistance to the development of cachexia in tumor-bearing mice. Int J Cancer 2010;126:756-63.
61. Schmitt TL, Martignoni ME, Bachmann J, Fechtner K, Friess H, Kinscherf R et al. Activity of the Akt-dependent anabolic and catabolic pathways in muscle and liver samples in cancer-related cachexia. J Mol Med (Berl) 2007; 85:647-54.
62. Pessina P, Conti V, Pacelli F, Rosa F, Doglietto GB, Brunelli S et al. Skeletal muscle of gastric cancer patients expresses genes involved in muscle regeneration. Oncol Rep 2010;24: 741-5.
63. He WA, Berardi E, Cardillo VM, Acharyya S, Aulino P, Thomas-Ahner J et al. NF-κB-mediated Pax7 dysregulation in the muscle microenvironment promotes cancer cachexia. J Clin Invest 2013;123:4821-35.
64. Argiles JM, Lopez-Soriano FJ. Catabolic pro-inflammatory citokines. Curr Opin Clin Nutr Metab Care 1998;1:245-51.
65. Cai D, Frantz JD, Tawa NE Jr, Melendez PA, Oh BC, Lidov HG et al. IKKbeta/NF-kappaB activation causes severe muscle wasting. Cell 2004;119:285-98.
66. Rhoads MG, Kandarian SC, Pacelli F, Doglietto GB, Bossola M. Expression of NF-kappaB and IkappaB proteins in skeletal muscle of gastric cancer patients. Eur J Cancer 2010;46: 191-7.
67. Llovera M, García-Martínez C, López-Soriano J, Carbó N, Agell N, López-Soriano FJ et al. Role of TNF receptor 1 in protein turnover during cancer cachexia using gene knockout mice. Mol Cell Endocrinol 1998;142:183-9.
68. Sishi BJ, Engelbrecht AM. Tumor necrosis factor alpha (TNF-α) inactivates the PI3-kinase/PKB pathway and induces atrophy and apoptosis in L6 myotubes. Cytokine 2011;54: 173-84.
69. Li YP, Chen Y, John J, Moylan J, Jin B, Mann DL et al. TNF-alpha acts via p38 MAPK to stimulate expression of the ubiquitin ligase atrogin1/MAFbx in skeletal muscle. FASEB J 2005;19:362-70.
70. Peterson JM, Bakkar N, Guttridge DC. NF-κB signaling in skeletal muscle health and disease. Curr Top Dev Biol 2011;96:85-119.
71. de Alvaro C, Teruel T, Hernandez R, Lorenzo M. Tumor necrosis factor alpha produces insulin resistance in skeletal muscle by activation of inhibitor kappaB kinase in a p38 MAPK-dependent manner. J Biol Chem 2004; 279:17070-8.
72. Guttridge DC, Mayo MW, Madrid LV, Wang CY, Baldwin AS Jr. NF-kappaB-induced loss of MyoD messenger RNA: possible role in muscle decay and cachexia. Science 2000;289: 2363-6.
73. Jatoi A, Ritter HL, Dueck A, Nguyen PL, Nikcevich DA, Luyun RF et al. A placebo-controlled, double-blind trial of infliximab for cancer-associated weight loss in elderly and/or poor performance non-small cell lung cancer patients (N01C9). Lung Cancer 2010;68: 234-9.
74. Strassmann G, Fong M, Kenney JS, Jacob CO. Evidence for the involvement of interleukin 6 in experimental cancer cachexia. J Clin Invest 1992; 89:1681-4.
75. Scott HR, McMillan DC, Crilly A, McArdle CS, Milroy R. The relationship between weight loss and interleukin 6 in non-small-cell lung cancer. Br J Cancer 1996;73:1560-2.
76. Seruga B, Zhang H, Bernstein LJ, Tannock IF. Cytokines and their relationship to the symptoms and outcome of cancer. Nat Rev Cancer 2008;8:887-99.
77. Moses AG, Maingay J, Sangster K, Fearon KC, Ross JA. Pro-inflammatory cytokine release by peripheral blood mononuclear cells from patients with advanced pancreatic cancer: relationship to acute phase response and survival. Oncol Rep 2009;21:1091-5.
78. Fischer P, Hilfiker-Kleiner D. Survival pathways in hypertrophy and heart failure: the gp130-STAT axis. Basic Res Cardiol 2007; 102:393-11.
79. Bonetto A, Aydogdu T, Jin X, Zhang Z, Zhan R, Puzis L et al. JAK/STAT3 pathway inhibition blocks skeletal muscle wasting downstream of IL-6 and in experimental cancer cachexia. Am J Physiol Endocrinol Metab 2012;303:E410-21.
80. Bayliss TJ, Smith JT, Schuster M, Dragnev

KH, Rigas JR. A humanized anti-IL-6 antibody (ALD518) in non-small cell lung cancer. Expert Opin Biol Ther 2011;11:1663-8.
81. Lee SJ, McPherron AC. Regulation of myostatin activity and muscle growth. Proc Natl Acad Sci USA 2001;98:9306-11.
82. Rebbapragada A, Benchabane H, Wrana JL, Celeste AJ, Attisano L. Myostatin signals through a transforming growth factor beta-like signaling pathway to block adipogenesis. Mol Cell Biol 2003; 23:7230-42.
83. Yang W, Chen Y, Zhang Y, Wang X, Yang N, Zhu D. Extracellular signal-regulated kinase 1/2 mitogen-activated protein kinase pathway is involved in myostatin-regulated differentiation repression. Cancer Res 2006;66:1320-6.
84. McFarlane C, Plummer E, Thomas M, Hennebry A, Ashby M, Ling N et al. Myostatin induces cachexia by activating the ubiquitin proteolytic system through an NF-kappaB-independent, FoxO1-dependent mechanism. J Cell Physiol 2006;209:501-14.
85. Benny Klimek ME, Aydogdu T, Link MJ, Pons M, Koniaris LG, Zimmers TA. Acute inhibition of myostatin-family proteins preserves skeletal muscle in mouse models of cancer cachexia. Biochem Biophys Res Commun 2010;391:1548-54.
86. Zhou X, Wang JL, Lu J, Song Y, Kwak KS, Jiao Q et al. Reversal of cancer cachexia and muscle wasting by ActRIIB antagonism leads to prolonged survival. Cell 2010;142:531-43.
87. Aversa Z, Bonetto A, Penna F, Costelli P, Di Rienzo G, Lacitignola A et al. Changes in myostatin signaling in non-weight-losing cancer patients. Ann Surg Oncol 2012;19:1350-6.
88. Dempsey DT, Knox LS, Mullen JL, Miller C, Feurer ID, Buzby GP. Energy expenditure in malnourished patients with colorectal cancer. Arch Surg 1986;121:789-95.
89. Gibney E, Elia M, Jebb SA, Murgatroyd P, Jennings G. Total energy expenditure in patients with small-cell lung cancer: results of a validated study using the bicarbonate-urea method. Metabolism 1997;46:1412-7.
90. Falconer JS, Fearon KC, Ross JA, Elton R, Wigmore SJ, Garden OJ et al. Acute-phase protein response and survival duration of patients with pancreatic cancer. Cancer 1995;75:2077-82.
91. Rossi Fanelli F, Cangiano C, Muscaritoli M, Conversano L, Torelli GF, Cascino A. Tumor-induced changes in host metabolism: a possible marker of neoplastic disease. Nutrition 1995;11(5 Suppl.):595-600.
92. Romanello V, Sandri M. Mitochondrial biogenesis and fragmentation as regulators of protein degradation in striated muscles. J Mol Cell Cardiol 2013;55:64-72.
93. White JP, Baltgalvis KA, Puppa MJ, Sato S, Baynes JW, Carson JA. Muscle oxidative capacity during IL-6-dependent cancer cachexia. Am J Physiol Regul Integr Comp Physiol 2011;300:R201-11.
94. Fontes-Oliveira CC, Busquets S, Toledo M, Penna F, Paz Aylwin M, Sirisi S et al. Mitochondrial and sarcoplasmic reticulum abnormalities in cancer cachexia: altered energetic efficiency? Biochim Biophys Acta 2013; 1830:2770-8.
95. Schiaffino S, Sandri M, Murgia M. Activity-dependent signaling pathways controlling muscle diversity and plasticity. Physiology (Bethesda) 2007; 22:269-78.
96. Brault JJ, Jespersen JG, Goldberg AL. Peroxisome proliferator-activated receptor gamma coactivator 1alpha or 1beta overexpression inhibits muscle protein degradation, induction of ubiquitin ligases, and disuse atrophy. J Biol Chem 2010;285:19460-71.
97. Sandri M, Lin J, Handschin C, Yang W, Arany ZP, Lecker SH et al. PGC-1alpha protects skeletal muscle from atrophy by suppressing FoxO3 action and atrophy-specific gene transcription. Proc Natl Acad Sci USA 2006;103:16260-5.
98. Wang X, Pickrell AM, Zimmers TA, Moraes CT. Increase in muscle mitochondrial biogenesis does not prevent muscle loss but increased tumor size in a mouse model of acute cancer-induced cachexia. PLoS One 2012;7:e33426.
99. Jäger S, Handschin C, St-Pierre J, Spiegelman BM. AMP-activated protein kinase (AMPK) action in skeletal muscle via direct phosphorylation of PGC-1alpha. Proc Natl Acad Sci USA 2007; 104:12017-22.
100. White JP, Puppa MJ, Gao S, Sato S, Welle SL, Carson JA. Muscle mTORC1 suppression by IL-6 during cancer cachexia: a role for AMPK. Am J Physiol Endocrinol Metab 2013;304: E1042-52.

ANOREXIA, REDUCED FOOD INTAKE AND SICKNESS BEHAVIOR IN CANCER CACHEXIA

A. MOLFINO, G. GIOIA, A. LAVIANO

INTRODUCTION

In recent years cancer anorexia-cachexia syndrome (CACS) was defined as the presence of reduced food intake, muscle and adipose tissue wasting, contributing to high morbidity, high mortality and reduced quality of life in cancer patients.[1] The prevalence of anorexia in cancer varies because factors other than treatment-induced effects, such as pain and depression, may reduce food intake. Cachexia is present in 2% of the general population but half of all cancer patients lose body weight. One third lose more than 5% of their body weight and up to 20% of all cancer deaths are related to cachexia. The incidence of weight loss upon diagnosis is influenced by the tumor site, with the greatest incidence of weight loss among patients affected by solid tumors, such as gastric, pancreatic, lung, colorectal, and head and neck. In the last 1-2 weeks of life, the overall prevalence of weight loss in cancer patients may increase to 86%.[2]

Anorexia is defined as the reduced or loss of desire to eat, and is a severely debilitating symptom throughout the clinical course of different chronic diseases (*i.e.* cancer, end-stage renal disease, chronic heart failure, chronic obstructive pulmonary disease, HIV/AIDS) that negatively impacts patient outcomes by contributing to weight loss, lean body mass and adipose tissue catabolism. Anorexia is now considered to be a component of the cachexia syndrome. Disease-associated anorexia is characterized by several symptoms, such as alterations in taste and smell, early satiety, meat aversion or nausea and vomiting, which are present even when calorie and protein intake is still preserved, in particular in the first disease phases.[3, 4] Malnutrition, anorexia and cachexia in cancer patients become more evident with tumor spread. Malnutrition is caused by mechanisms linked to the primary tumor or damage by specific anticancer therapies such as surgery, chemotherapy, radiotherapy. Anorexia is associated with meal-related neural and humoral signals related to body fat or energy storage interacting with the hypothalamus and determining hypothalamic altered response. The sickness behavior syndrome is a disease adaptive reaction resulting in the release of proinflammatory cytokines (interleukin-1, interleukin-6, and tumor necrosis factor-α) from the immune response, and consists of several symptoms such as lethargy, depression, reduced food intake, fever, anhedonia, cognitive impairment, hyperalgesia, and decreased social interaction. Sickness behavior in cancer patients results from both the presence of the disease and the side effects of the anticancer treatments, and sickness behavior-related cytokine release may explain several cancer-related symptoms, including anorexia.[5] Sickness behavior can also be related to depressive symptoms that should be always investigated.

PATHOGENIC MECHANISMS

The pathogenesis of anorexia and cachexia is multifactorial and is determined by alterations of the central physiological mechanisms modulating energy intake. Mediators regulate food intake involving links between neuropeptides and neurotransmitters in the central nervous system (CNS).[6] Several symptoms, including meat aversion, and taste and smell alterations, might be directly related to alterations in the neuroendocrine pathways. Short-term acting mediators, peptides produced by enteroendocrine system, account for satiety signals by acting through the bloodstream or the vagus nerve on the CNS.[4]

The response of the endocrine pancreas to nutrients is improved by the incretin hormones glucagon-like-peptide 1 (GLP-1), glucose-dependent insulinotropic polypeptide (GIP), and potentially oxyntomodulin (OXM). In particular, GLP-1 and OXM reduce food intake and ghrelin, released by the stomach, stimulates appetite. Within the hormones promoting satiety, cholecystokinin (CCK), pancreatic polypeptide (PP), peptide tyrosine-tyrosine (PYY), and OXM, play a major role. Hormonal signals represent long-term acting mediators and are mainly represented by leptin, adiponectin, and insulin. The storage of absorbed nutrients and energy balance is regulated by insulin, also acting as an adiposity signal to the brain. Leptin informs the brain of adipose energy storage by binding to specific receptors on appetite-modulating neurons in the arcuate nucleus. Low leptin levels increase the hypothalamic orexigenic signals stimulating food assumption and reducing anorexigenic symptoms.[7,8]

The hypothalamus physiologically plays a role in the control of food intake and energy expenditure by transducing peripheral signals into neuronal activities. The arcuate nucleus, which is situated between the third ventricle and the median eminence, is the most important hypothalamic area regulating energy expenditure.[9] Two different neuronal cells in the arcuate nucleus regulate energy balance. The first subset of neurons co-expresses proopiomelanocortin (POMC), a precursor molecule that is cleaved into peptides named melanocortins, and cocaine-and amphetamine-regulated transcript (CART), promoting anorexigenic effects. POMC stimulates the anorectic peptide α-melanocyte-stimulating hormone (α-MSH), an agonist at the melanocortin-3 (MC3R) and melanocortin-4 (MC4R) receptors. The second subset of neurons synthesizes neuropeptide Y (NPY), promoting food intake, feeding, and agouti-related protein (AgRP) that also increases appetite.[10,11] AgRP is an endogenous antagonist of MC3R and MC4R and its administration in experimental model was associated with increased food intake. Hypothalamic neurons responding to peripheral signals influence synthesis of neuropeptides. From the periphery, ghrelin, produced mainly by the stomach, stimulates NPY/AgRP neurons and inhibits the expression of POMC, thereby stimulating feeding and inhibiting energy expenditure. Leptin regulates fat storage, activates POMC/CART neurons, and inhibits NPY/AgRP neurons, reducing food intake and enhancing energy expenditure.

Insulin inhibits the orexigenic NPY/AgRP neurons thus downregulating food intake.[12] In the presence of cancer-associated anorexia and cachexia, leptin levels are reduced, whereas ghrelin concentrations are elevated or normal.[13,14] The continuous activation of POMC neurons determines a hypothalamic deranged response to signals from the periphery. The melanocortin system is hyper-activated in cancer anorexia and cachexia.[15]

IL-1β administered directly into the brain antagonizes NPY-induced feeding in anorectic tumor-bearing rats, decreasing hypothalamic specific NPY mRNA levels.[16] These results support the idea that the NPY system is altered in anorexia induced by IL-1β.[16]

The hypothalamic neurotransmitter serotonin, synthesized from tryptophan, contributes to satiety regulation by depressing food intake. Plasma and cerebrospinal fluid levels of tryptophan are increased in the course of cancer-associated anorexia and more tryptophan goes to the central nervous system and, in parallel, more serotonin is released. Peripheral infusion of IL-1 induces anorexia and raises brain tryptophan levels, suggesting increased serotonin synthesis.[17] During the catabolic state, increased hypothalamic expression of IL-1 is associated with a higher concentration of serotonin levels. IL-1 and serotonin act within the ARC nucleus conditioning the melanocortin system, inhibiting the NPY/AgRP system, and inducing the suppression of the inhibition of POMC neurons thus enhancing the release of the α-MSH, which is the MC4R agonist, and reducing the release of the AgRP, which is the MC4R antagonist.[17] Cancer anorexia is strictly related to the presence of inflammation. Experimental evidence demonstrated that the administration of different cytokines, such as IL-1-α, IL-1-β, TNF-α, increased the production of leptin thus inhibiting food intake and preventing the physiological compensatory mechanisms against the presence of anorexia.[18] Prostaglandins also have been shown to be involved in experimental models of anorexia.[19] In this light, therapeutic strategies aimed at interfering with prostaglandin synthesis lead to favorable clinical effects.[20] A role in the pathogenesis of cancer anorexia is also played by substances produced directly by the tumors, such as macrophage inhibitory cytokine-1 (MIC-1).[21]

DIAGNOSIS AND ASSESSMENT OF CANCER ANOREXIA

The presence of anorexia can be identified by the use of specific questionnaires. Visual analog scales, either anchored or not anchored, are also often used to objectively quantify severity (the degree of anorexia) and appetite loss, but may not detect small changes in appetite.[23] The use of questionnaires provides a qualitative assessment of the presence of anorexia, identifying patients at higher risk of complications in different clinical settings. Questionnaires that provide both qualitative and quantitative assessment of cancer anorexia are mainly based on a comprehensive assessment of appetite and appetite-related symptoms such as the Functional Assessment of Anorexia/Cachexia Therapy (FAACT) questionnaire and the North Central Cancer Treatment Group (NCCTG) Anorexia/Cachexia questionnaire. The FAACT questionnaire (Tab. 4-I), used

Table 4-I – Symptom-based assessment of anorexia (adapted from reference [23]).					
	Not at all	A little bit	Somewhat	Quite a bit	Very much
I have a good appetite	0	1	1	3	4
The amount I eat is sufficient to meet my needs	0	1	1	3	4
I am worried about my weight	0	1	2	3	4
Most food tastes unpleasant to me	4	3	2	1	0
I am concerned about how thin I look	4	3	2	1	0
My interest in food drops as soon as I try to eat	4	3	2	1	0
I have difficulty eating rich or "heavy" foods	4	3	2	1	0
My family or friends are pressuring me to eat	4	3	2	1	0
I have been vomiting	4	3	2	1	0
When I eat, I seem to get fully quickly	4	3	2	1	0
I have pain in my stomach area	4	3	2	1	0
My general health is improving	0	1	2	3	4

Table 4-I Symptoms negatively affecting food intake and directly related to modifications in the central nervous system regulating energy intake. Patients affected by at least one of these symptoms can be defined as anorexic.

Symptoms
Early satiety
Taste alterations
Smell alterations
Meat aversion
Nausea/vomiting

to test the efficacy of anti-anorexia/cachexia therapies, is divided into five sections and includes 39 items, 12 of which are related to nutritional issues. It is a useful clinical scale to identify general aspects of the quality of life related to cancer anorexia and cachexia, and it is a modification of the "Functional Assessment of Anorexia-Cachexia Therapy-General" scale. The NCCTG Anorexia/Cachexia questionnaire includes 15 items, 10 of which related to nutritional issues.[24, 25] We also know of a symptom-based questionnaire (Tab. 4-II) that is able to identify patients with deteriorated nutritional status and likely altered brain neurochemistry which leads to deranged control of eating behavior, but more studies are needed to strengthen the reliability of this questionnaire in identifying anorexic patients. This questionnaire is particularly aimed at identifying the presence of early satiety, taste and/or smell alterations and nausea. Finally, the Malnutrition Screening Tool (MST) and Patient-Generated Subjective Global Assessment of Nutritional Status (PG-SGA) are useful validated evaluation instruments in the diagnosis of nutritional risk and cancer anorexia.[26-28]

THE TREATMENT OF CANCER ANOREXIA

The treatment of cancer anorexia is based on nutritional support and pharmacological treatment. Nutritional treatment includes dietary counseling (fractioned intake, food chosen according to the patient's ability to swallow, avoiding strong smells), nutritional supplements and artificial nutrition. Nutritional supplements increase protein and calorie intake (including products enriched with ω-3 fatty acids considering their anti-inflammatory properties).[29]

The pharmacological treatment of anorexia is aimed at the modulation of cytokines, hormones or the different catabolic or anabolic metabolic pathways. Specific molecules will be analyzed in the chapter dedicated to pharmacological strategies in treating cancer cachexia.

CONCLUSIONS

Anorexia, reduced food intake and sickness behavior negatively impact morbidity and mortality in cancer patients. Its pathogenesis recognizes multiple mechanisms. Anorexia is mainly due to hypothalamic dysfunction and its treatment involves pharmaceutical and nutritional interventions, but we need more research and clinical trials to recognize the efficacy of the use of different molecules. One future research line is to combine different pharmacological treatments for cancer anorexia to act on different pathophysiological mechanisms at the same time, to improve appetite.

BIBLIOGRAFIA

1. Bennani-Baiti N, Walsh D. What is cancer anorexia-cachexia syndrome? A historical perspective. J R Coll Physicians Edinb 2009;39:257-62.
2. Tan BH, Fearon KC. Cachexia: prevalence and impact in medicine. Curr Opin Clin Nutr Metab Care 2008;11:400-7.
3. Molfino A, Laviano A, Rossi Fanelli F. Contribution of anorexia to tissue wasting in cachexia. Curr Opin Support Palliat Care 2010;4:249-53.
4. Nicolini A, Ferrari P, Masoni MC, Fini M, Pagani S, Giampietro O *et al*. Malnutrition, anorexia and cachexia in cancer patients: A mini-review on pathogenesis and treatment. Biomed Pharmacother 2013;67:807-17.

5. Myers JS. Proinflammatory cytokines and sickness behavior: implications for depression and cancer-related symptoms. Oncol Nurs Forum 2008;35:802-7.
6. Rolls ET. Taste, olfactory, and food texture processing in the brain, and the control of food intake. Physiol Behav 2005;85:45-56.
7. Berthoud HR. Neural control of appetite: cross-talk between homeostatic and non homeostatic systems. Appetite 2004;43:315-7.
8. Inui A. Feeding and body-weight regulation by hypothalamic neuropeptides-mediation of the actions of leptin. Trends Neurosci 1999;22:62-7.
9. Laviano A, Inui A, Marks DL, Meguid MM, Pichard C, Rossi Fanelli F et al. Neural control of the anorexia-cachexia syndrome. Am J Physiol Endocrinol Metab 2008;295:E1000-8.
10. Abdel-Malek ZA. Melanocortin receptors: their functions and regulation by physiological agonists and antagonists. Cell Mol Life Sci 2001;58:434-41.
11. Lu XY, Nicholson JR, Akil H, Watson SJ. Time course of short-term and long-term orexigenic effects of agouti-related protein (86-132). Neuroreport 2001;12:1281-4.
12. Morton GJ, Cummings DE, Baskin DG, Barsh GS, Schwartz MW. Central nervous system control of food intake and body weight. Nature 2006;443:289-95.
13. Mantovani G, Macciò A, Mura L, Massa E, Mudu MC, Mulas C et al. Serum levels of leptin and proinflammatory cytokines in patients with advanced-stage cancer at different sites. J Mol Med 2000;78:554-61.
14. Inui A, Asakawa A, Bowers CY, Mantovani G, Laviano A, Meguid MM et al. Ghrelin, appetite, and gastric motility: the emerging role of the stomach as an endocrine organ. FASEB J 2004;18:439-56.
15. Ellacott KL, Cone RD. The central melanocortin system and the integration of short- and long-term regulators of energy homeostasis. Recent Prog Horm Res 2004;59:395-408.
16. Inui A. Neuropeptide Y. A key molecule in anorexia and cachexia in wasting disorders. Mol Med Today 1999;5:79-85.
17. Kaye WH, Frank GK, Bailer UF, Henry SE, Meltzer CC, Price JC et al. Serotonin alterations in anorexia and bulimia nervosa: new insights from imaging studies. Physiol Behav 2005;85:73-81.
18. Sato T, Laviano A, Meguid MM, Chen C, Rossi-Fanelli F, Hatakeyama K. Involvement of plasma leptin, insulin and free tryptophan in cytokine-induced anorexia. Clin Nutr 2003;22:139-46.
19. Wang W, Andersson M, Lonnroth C, Svanberg E, Lundholm K. Prostaglandin E and prostacyclin receptor expression in tumor and host tissues from MCG 101-bearing mice: a model with prostanoid-related cachexia. Int J Cancer 2005;115:582-90.
20. Lundholm K, Daneryd P, Bosaeus I, Körner U, Lindholm E. Palliative nutritional intervention in addition to cyclooxygenase and erythropoietin treatment for patients with malignant disease: Effects on survival, metabolism, and function. Cancer 2004;100:1967-77.
21. Johnen H, Lin S, Kuffner T, Brown DA, Tsai VW, Bauskin AR et al. Tumor induced anorexia and weight loss are mediated by the TGF-beta superfamily cytokine MIC-1. Nat Med 2007;13:1333-40.
22. Stubbs RJ, Hughes DA, Johnstone AM, Rowley E, Reid C, Elia M et al. The use of visual analogue scales to assess motivation to eat in human subjects: a review of their reliability and validity with an evaluation of new hand-held computerized systems for temporal tracking of appetite ratings. Br J Nutr 2000;84:405-15.
23. Ribaudo JM, Cella D, Hahn EA, Lloyd SR, Tchekmedyian NS, Von Roenn J et al. Re-validation and shortening of the Functional Assessment of Anorexia/ Cachexia Therapy (FAACT) questionnaire. Qual Life Res 2000;9:1137-46.
24. National Institute of Health. Interactive Textbook on Clinical Symptom Research. Available at: http://symptomresearch.nih.gov.
25. Walsh D, Rybicki L, Nelson KA, Donnelly S. Symptoms and prognosis in advanced cancer. Support Care Cancer 2002;10:385-8.
26. Kubrak C, Jensen L. Critical evaluation of nutrition screening tools recommended for oncology patients. Cancer Nursing 2007;30:E1-6.
27. Isenring E, Cross G, Daniels L, Kellett E, Koczwara B. Validity of the malnutrition screening tool as an effective predictor of nutritional risk in oncology outpatients receiving chemotherapy. Support Care Cancer 2006;14:152-6.
28. Mantovani G, Madeddu C. Cancer cachexia: medical management. Support Care Cancer 2010;18:1-9.

PHARMACOLOGIC THERAPY OF CACHEXIA

A. LAVIANO, S. RIANDA, A. MARI

INTRODUCTION

As outlined in the previous chapters of this book, wasting is a frequent and complex problem in cancer patients. The pathogenesis of cancer cachexia is related to the combined effects of different factors, including anorexia, gastrointestinal (GI) dysfunction, systemic inflammatory response and increased release of catabolic signals (Tab. 5-I). Many different pharmacologic approaches have been proposed to treat the components of the cachexia network (Tab. 5-II), but only a few have so far been proven effective. It is important to highlight that physical activity is key to promoting muscle anabolism, and therefore, any pharmacological treatment in cancer patients should necessarily be combined with exercise training.

Table 5-I – Catabolic factors.

Dysfunction	Treatment
Anorexia	Appetite stimulants
Gastrointestinal dysfunction	GI modulators and other supportive agents
Systemic inflammation	Anti-inflammatory agents
Catabolism	Anticatabolic and anabolic agents

Table 5-II – Pharmacologic approaches to treat cachexia.

Appetite stimulants	Gastrointestinal modulators and other supportive agents	Anti-inflammatory agents	Anti-catabolic and anabolic agents
Corticosteroids	Prokinetic drugs	Steroids, cannabinoids	Insulin and insulin sensitivity modulators
Progestins	Inhibitors of GI motility	NSAID	Growth hormone and secretagogues
Cannabinoids	Proton pump inhibitors	N-3 fatty acids	Anabolic-androgenic steroids and SARMs
Ghrelin and analogues	Parasympathomimetics	Anti-interleukin 6 antibodies	Amino acids, metabolites
Melanocortin 4 receptor antagonists	Anti-emetics	Anti-cytokine agents	Experimental agents (anti-myostatin, selumetinib, IL 15)
Cyproheptadine	Analgesics	Antibiotics (clarithromycin)	Proteasome inhibitors
BCAA	Psychotropic drugs	Melatonin	ß-receptor modulators
Herbal medicine, bitters		Antioxidants	Hydrazine sulfate
			ATP

BCAA: branched-chain amino acids. NSAID: non-steroidal anti-inflammatory drug. SARM: selective androgen receptor modulator. ATP: adenosine 5′-triphosphate

TREATMENT OF CANCER CACHEXIA

Table 5-III – Agents tested to treat anorexia.
Appetite stimulants
Corticosteroids
Progestins
Cannabinoids
Ghrelin and analogues
Melanocortin 4 receptor antagonists
Cyproheptadine
Branched-chain amino acids
Herbal medicines, bitters

APPETITE STIMULANTS

Anorexia is frequently observed in cancer patients and impinges on the QoL of patients and their families. It also has a negative impact on clinical outcomes.[1] A number of agents have been tested to treat anorexia and increase appetite (Tab. 5-III).

Corticosteroids (dexamethasone, prednisolone, methylprednisolone and hydrocortisone). These agents stimulate appetite and involve antiemetic activity. These effects are achieved by the suppression of the production or release of proinflammatory cytokines, and usually last only a few weeks.

Many trials have shown that intravenous or oral corticosteroids significantly improve appetite, pain, QoL, vomiting and well-being,[2] however, beneficial effects disappeared after four weeks. Adverse effects of long-term corticosteroid therapy include myopathy, osteoporosis, immune suppression, susceptibility to infections, skin frailty, accumulation of extracellular water, edema, insulin resistance and hyperglycemia, GI ulcers and mood abnormalities.

Progestins [megestrol acetate (MA) and medroxyprogesterone acetate (MPA)]. MA at doses from 160 to 1600 mg/d and MPA at doses from 300 to 1200 mg/d improved appetite and, less reliably, body weight, while there were only minimal effects on QoL.[2, 3] A more recent meta-analysis[4] concluded that MA reduces the symptoms of cancer cachexia with no effect on survival or QoL. Unfortunately, weight gain is not generally accompanied by an increase in lean body mass.[5] Side effects of progestins include thromboembolism,[6] impotence in males and vaginal spotting or bleeding in females, hyperglycemia, hypertension, peripheral edema, alopecia, and adrenal insufficiency.

Cannabinoids [tetrahydrocannabinol (THC)]. Cannabinoids bind to the receptors of the endocannabinoid system in the central nervous system. Side effects are not uncommon, including nausea and slurred speech. A recent trial[7] did not show any benefit of oral administration of cannabis extract or THC.

Ghrelin and analogues (experimental agents). Ghrelin is a peptide hormone mainly produced in the stomach, which stimulates food intake and adiposity. Small trials suggest that ghrelin improves appetite and food intake, but no effects on muscularity have been consistently reported.[8-11]

The orally active growth hormone secretagogue receptor agonist anamorelin (RC-1291) has been shown to produce an increase in body mass and grip strength and a trend towards increased lean mass but no benefit to quality of life.[12]

Melanocortin 4 receptor (MC4R) antagonists (experimental agents): the hypothalamic melanocortin system mediates the onset of anorexia, increased energy expenditure and loss of lean body mass through MC4 receptors. Antagonists for MC4R are being developed and tested to inhibit inflammation-associated anorexia.[13] Only preclinical data has been so far obtained.

Cyproheptadine. Cyproheptadine is a serotonin antagonist acting as a 5-HT$_2$ receptor antagonist. A randomized double-blind trial in cancer patients with anorexia or cachexia failed to prevent weight loss compared with the placebo group.[14]

Branched-chain amino acids (BCAA). It has been proposed that increased hypothalamic serotonergic activity might play a role in the development of anorexia.[1] Since BCAA competes with tryptophan for the same transport system across the blood-brain barrier, it has been suggested that BCAA might reduce the brain entry of tryptophan, which in turn leads to decreased brain tryptophan concentration and reduced serotoninergic activity and finally decreased anorexia. Two small randomized controlled studies (RCTs) tested this hypothesis in cancer patients, with positive results.[15, 16]

Herbal medicines, bitters. Herbal bitters and other herbal remedies have been used in many countries to increase or stabilize appetite.[17] Clinical evidence to support the use of herbal medicine is very sparse and does not allow its recommendation.

GASTROINTESTINAL MODULATORS AND OTHER SUPPORTIVE AGENTS

Anti-emetics, psychotropic drugs and analgesics may alleviate nausea and emesis, anxiety, restlessness and depression, or chronic pain in cancer patients. Since these symptoms invariably diminish or abolish appetite and food intake, it is of considerable importance that clinical nutritionists actively investigate their presence.

GI functions are key for food intake, propulsion, digestion and absorption. Dysfunction or defects may prevent the adequate uptake of energy and nutrients. Modulators of GI function may thus help to antagonize weight loss in cancer patients (Tab. 5-IV).

Table 5-IV – Agents enhancing GI function.

Gastrointestinal modulators and other supportive agents
Anti-emetics
Psychotropic drugs
Analgesics
Prokinetic agents
Inhibitors of GI motility
Proton pump inhibitors
Parasympathomimetics

Prokinetic agents. Metoclopramide (80 mg/d) improves nausea but does not increase caloric intake or appetite. Erythromycin improves delayed gastric emptying.[18]

Inhibitors of gastrointestinal motility. Chemotherapy-induced diarrhea leads to weight loss and dehydration. Inhibition of intestinal transit time may diminish diarrhea by increasing the time for reabsorption of secreted intestinal fluids. Typical agents used are opioids, calcium channel blockers, and clonidine.

Proton pump inhibitors. Drugs frequently used in cancer patients increase the occurrence of GI ulceration, which may lead to abdominal pain, nausea, vomiting, anorexia and weight loss. Inhibition of gastric acid secretion is an effective way to allow the healing of ulcerations. Proton pump inhibitors are the most powerful drugs available to achieve this end.

Parasympathomimetic. Many drugs, as well as radiotherapy to the head and neck region, may cause dry mouth (xerostomia). Pilocarpine is a parasympathomimetic plant alkaloid, which stimulates the secretion of large amounts of saliva and sweat. This may help to increase appetite and achieve improved conditions for chewing and swallowing.

Table 5-V – Modulation of inflammatory response.
Anti-inflammatory agents
Corticosteroids, progestins, cannabinoids
NSAID
N-3 fatty acids
Anti-interleukin 6 antibodies
Anti-cytokine agents
Antibiotics (clarithromycin)
Melatonin
Antioxidants

ANTI-INFLAMMATORY AGENTS

Systemic inflammation is a frequent and prognostically relevant phenomenon in patients with advanced cancer.[19] A large number of anti-inflammatory agents have been studied (Tab. 5-V).

Steroids (corticosteroids and progestins) and cannabinoids. This topic has been addressed in previous sections of this chapter.

Non-steroidal anti-inflammatory drugs (NSAID). NSAIDs such as indomethacin, ibuprofen and celecoxib inhibit prostaglandin production via the rate-limiting enzymes cyclooxygenases-1 and -2 (COX-1 and COX-2). COX-2 is induced by cytokines, growth factors, and oncogenes. Indomethacin (100 mg/d) prolongs mean survival time.[20] Ibuprofen (1200 mg/d) reduces elevated resting energy expenditure and C-reactive protein levels.[21] Mantovani et al.[22] studied the efficacy and safety of celecoxib (300 mg/d) and reported significant improvements in lean body mass, grip strength, quality of life and performance status. In a systematic review, Solheim et al. evaluated 13 clinical studies using NSAIDs to treat cancer cachexia[23] and concluded that NSAIDs may improve weight in cancer patients with cachexia but that evidence is too frail to recommend these drugs for the treatment of cachexia outside clinical trials.

Omega-3 fatty acids (EPA, DHA). Fish oil is particularly rich in long-chain N-3 polyunsaturated fatty acids including eicosapentaenoic (EPA; C20:5; n-3) and docosahexaenoic (DHA; C22:6; n-3) acids. These undergo biological transformation by COX to produce eicosanoids, which alters the production of inflammatory mediators, including cytokines. EPA is a competitive antagonist of arachidonic acid and is transformed to less pro-inflammatory eicosanoids. EPA may thus decrease inflammatory status.

Several RCTs have studied the effects of N-3 fatty acids on cancer cachexia.[24-28] While well designed clinical trials reporting on the effects of n-3 fatty acids on clinical outcome in cachectic cancer patients are lacking, the results of these recent trials are promising. Side effects of fish oil and n-3 fatty acids are small. The decision to recommend supplements of n-3 fatty acids needs to be made on an individual basis.

Anti-interleukin 6 antibodies (experimental agents). Interleukin 6 (IL-6) is a major mediator of the acute phase response. IL-6 is associated with poor prognosis in patients with lung cancer and correlates to symptoms such as fatigue and cachexia.[29] Only Phase I and II trials, and anecdotal reports have so far been published,[29-31] and therefore no general recommendation can be made.

Anti-cytokine agents. Pro-inflammatory cytokines mediate many of the metabolic derangements observed in cancer cachexia.[32-34] Different strategies to suppress or block cytokines have been developed, including TNF-binding agents,[35, 36] pentoxifylline,[37] and thalidomide,[38] with uncertain results.

Antibiotics (Clarithromycin). Limited and inconclusive evidence to support its use.

Melatonin. Melatonin (N-acetyl-5-methoxytryptamine) is secreted into the blood by the pineal gland in a diurnal rhythm. It has powerful antioxidant effects. Confirmatory reports in cancer patients are still lacking, and therefore melatonin has not entered standard treatment protocols.

Antioxidants. No reliable randomized studies have been published to judge the effect of antioxidants in cancer.

ANTICATABOLIC AND ANABOLIC AGENTS

A number of endogenous and exogenous agents are being used or investigated to inhibit proteolysis or to stimulate protein synthesis (Tab. 5-VI).

Insulin and insulin sensitivity modulators. Daily insulin treatment (0.11 IU/kg/d) integrating basic supportive care increases whole body fat (but not lean body mass), improves metabolic efficiency during exercise (but not maximum exercise capacity or spontaneous physical activity) and improves overall survival.[39]

Growth hormone (GH), GH secretagogues and insulin-like growth factor 1 (IGF-1). There is concern regarding the use of GH because of the possible stimulation of tumor growth. Preclinical data have not shown tumor progression,[40] however valid clinical data are lacking.

Ghrelin is a GH secretagogue. For ghrelin see the previous section in this chapter. IGF-1 is an anabolic hormone similar in structure to insulin. Recently, IGF-1 has been linked to tumor development and progression.[41]

Anabolic-androgenic steroids. Anabolic steroids or anabolic-androgenic steroids (AAS) are drugs which mimic the effects of testosterone and dihydrotestosterone. They increase protein synthesis within cells, especially in muscles. Anabolic steroids also have an-

Table 5-VI – Modulation of protein metabolism.
Anti-catabolic and anabolic agents
Insulin and insulin sensitivity modulators
Growth hormone, GH secretagogues, IGF-1
Anabolic-androgenic steroids and SARMs
Amino acids and metabolites
Anti-myostatin antibodies
Selumetinib
Interleukin 15
Proteasome inhibitors
ß-receptor modulators
Hydrazine sulfate
Adenosine 5'-triphosphate

drogenic and virilizing properties. In patients with advanced cancer, decreased free testosterone levels are frequently observed. Use of nandrolone decanoate (200 mg/week) resulted in less weight loss.[42] Fluoxymesterone (20 m/d) resulted in less appetite stimulation than other anti-cachexia agents.[6] Patients treated with oxandrolone still lost weight but experienced an increase in lean body mass, a reduction in fat mass and reduced self-reported anorectic symptoms.[5]

Selective androgen receptor modulators (SARMs) have been developed for the treatment of muscle wasting and osteoporosis. The oral SARM enobosarm resulted in improved lean body mass and muscle function.[43] Preliminary results are emerging and show that enobosarm resulted in better maintenance/improvement of LBM and in better muscle function (measured as stair climbing power) than a placebo.

Amino acids and metabolites. In-vitro and *in-vivo* studies have demonstrated the anti-catabolic effects of leucine and its metabolites α-ketoisocaproate and the ketone body ß-hydroxy ß-methylbutyrate (HMB). There is accumulating evidence that protein and especially leucine and its metabolite HMB may support muscle mass by increasing synthetic rate and/or decreasing protein breakdown. Even though these mechanisms appear plausible, more solid evidence from high-quality studies with cancer patients is required before the use of leucine and HMB can be generally recommended.

Experimental agents:
- *Anti-myostatin antibodies*; myostatin is a member of the transforming growth factor-ß superfamily and downregulates skeletal muscle mass by binding to the activin A receptor IIB (Act RIIB). Myostatin levels are increased in tumor-bearing rats and thus might be a therapeutic target in cancer cachexia.[44] In a mouse model, injection of the myostatin binding soluble Act RIIB after tumor cell implantation resulted in a reversal of tumor-induced weight loss and improved survival.
- *Selumetinib*; induction of muscle anabolism by physical activity occurs along pathways involving RAF, MEK and MAPK/ERK kinases.[45] The anti-cancer agent selumetinib is a MEK inhibitor, has tumor suppressive activity and has been shown to inhibit IL-6 production. In a phase II trial, retrospective analysis of skeletal muscle mass demonstrated that patients with cholangiocellular carcinoma gained muscle mass when treated with selumetinib.[45] Further investigation of these beneficial effects is required.
- *Interleukin 15*; the cytokine IL-15 shares biological activities with IL-2 but is not produced by activated T cells, but by skeletal muscle, kidney, lung and heart. IL-15 favors muscle fiber hypertrophy and partly inhibits muscle wasting in tumor-bearing rats.[46] IL-15 stimulates protein synthesis and inhibits protein degradation.[47] No clinical trials using IL-15 have been reported.
- *Proteasome inhibitors* (Bortezomib); bortezomib is an inhibitor of NFkB and ubiquitin-proteasome. Although potentially promising, preliminary results showed negligible effects from these molecules on cancer-related weight loss in patients with metastatic pancreatic cancer.[48]
- *ß-Adrenergic receptor modulators*; ß-Adrenergic receptors are involved in anabolic signaling and modulation of resting energy expenditure.[49] Hyltander et al.[50] reported that treatment with a selective ß1- (atenolol) as well as with a non-specific ß1,ß2-adrenoreceptor (propranolol) antagonist reduced resting energy expenditure in weight losing cancer patients. Part of this reduction was explained by a decline in heart rate. Administration of the ß2-agonist formoterol to both rats and mice bearing highly cachectic tumors resulted in a reversal of the muscle wasting process.[51] Recently, in a small group of patients with cancer cachexia, intake of formoterol in combination with the progestin MA for eight weeks resulted in an increase in quadriceps and hand grip strength.[52]
- *Hydrazine sulfate*; hydrazine is a non-competitive inhibitor of phosphoenolpyruvate carboxykinase, one of the enzymes needed for gluconeogenesis. Gold proposed that inhibiting gluconeogenesis in cancer patients would reduce their energy loss and thus development of cachexia,[53] however, clinical trials reported a trend for poorer survival [54, 55] and significantly worse quality of life in the hydrazine group. Hydrazine is not recommended for treatment of anorexia or cachexia.
- *Adenosine 5'-triphosphate (ATP)*; adenosine 5'-triphosphate is a naturally occurring nucleoside triphosphate that plays a central role as an energy source in every cell of the human body. Small clinical trials showed that ATP infusion in weight losing cancer patients stabilized body weight,[56] improved triceps skinfold thickness,[57] but had no effect on quality of life, functional

status or fatigue.[58] In addition, overall survival was significant longer in weight losing cancer patients receiving ATP.[59] ATP is a promising agent but is not recommended outside clinical trials.

REFERENCES

1. Laviano A, Meguid MM, Inui A, Muscaritoli M, Rossi Fanelli F. Therapy insight: Cancer anorexia-cachexia syndrome - When all you can eat is yourself. Nat Clin Pract Oncol 2005;2:158-65.
2. Yavuzsen T, Davis MP, Walsh D, LeGrand S, Lagman R. Systematic review of the treatment of cancer-associated anorexia and weight loss. J Clin Oncol 2005;23:8500-11.
3. Berenstein EG, Ortiz Z. Megestrol acetate for the treatment of anorexia-cachexia syndrome. Cochrane Database Syst Rev 2005;CD004310.
4. Leśniak W, Bała M, Jaeschke R, Krzakowski M. Effects of megestrol acetate in patients with cancer anorexia-cachexia syndrome--a systematic review and meta-analysis. Pol Arch Med Wewn 2008;118:636-44.
5. Lesser G, Case D, Ottery F, McQuellon R, Choksi J, Sanders G et al. A phase III randomized study comparing the effects of oxandrolone and megestrolacetate on lean body mass, weight and quality of life in patients with solid tumors and weight loss receiving chemotherapy. In: ASCO 2008. Alexandria, Va: 2008. p. Abstract 9513.
6. Loprinzi CL, Kugler JW, Sloan JA, Mailliard JA, Krook JE, Wilwerding MB et al. Randomized comparison of megestrol acetate versus dexamethasone versus fluoxymesterone for the treatment of cancer anorexia/cachexia. J Clin Oncol 1999;17:3299-306.
7. Strasser F, Luftner D, Possinger K, Ernst G, Ruhstaller T, Meissner W et al. Comparison of orally administered cannabis extract and delta-9-tetrahydrocannabinol in treating patients with cancer-related anorexia-cachexia syndrome: a multicenter, phase III, randomized, double-blind, placebo-controlled clinical trial from the Cannabis-In-Cachexia-Study-Group. J Clin Oncol 2006;24:3394-400.
8. Neary NM, Small CJ, Wren AM, Lee JL, Druce MR, Palmieri C et al. Ghrelin increases energy intake in cancer patients with impaired appetite: acute, randomized, placebo-controlled trial. J Clin Endocrinol Metab 2004;89:2832-6.
9. Strasser F, Lutz TA, Maeder MT, Thuerlimann B, Bueche D, Tschöp M et al. Safety, tolerability and pharmacokinetics of intravenous ghrelin for cancer-related anorexia/cachexia: a randomised, placebo-controlled, double-blind, double-crossover study. Br J Cancer 2008;98: 300-8.
10. Adachi S, Takiguchi S, Okada K, Yamamoto K, Yamasaki M, Miyata H et al. Effects of ghrelin administration after total gastrectomy: a prospective, randomized, placebo-controlled phase II study. Gastroenterology 2010;138:1312-20.
11. Lundholm K, Gunnebo L, Körner U, Iresjö B-M, Engström C, Hyltander A et al. Effects by daily long term provision of ghrelin to unselected weight-losing cancer patients: a randomized double-blind study. Cancer 2010;116:2044-52.
12. Garcia J, Boccia R, Graham C, Kumor K, Polvino W. A phase II randomized, placebo-controlled, double-blind study of the efficacy and safety of RC-1291 (RC) for the treatment of cancer cachexia. In: ASCO 2007. Alexandria, Va: 2007. p. Abstract 9133.
13. Tran JA, Tucci FC, Jiang W, Marinkovic D, Chen CW, Arellano M et al. Pyrrolidinones as orally bioavailable antagonists of the human melanocortin-4 receptor with anti-cachectic activity. Bioorg Med Chem 2007;15:5166-76.
14. Kardinal CG, Loprinzi CL, Schaid DJ, Hass AC, Dose AM, Athmann LM et al. A controlled trial of cyproheptadine in cancer patients with anorexia and/or cachexia. Cancer 1990;65:2657-62.
15. Cangiano C, Laviano A, Meguid MM, Mulieri M, Conversano L, Preziosa I et al. Effects of administration of oral branched-chain amino acids on anorexia and caloric intake in cancer patients. J Natl Cancer Inst 1996;88:550-2.
16. Poon RT-P, Yu W-C, Fan S-T, Wong J. Long-term oral branched chain amino acids in patients undergoing chemoembolization for hepatocellular carcinoma: a randomized trial. Aliment Pharmacol Ther 2004;19:779-88.
17. Cheng K-C, Li Y-X, Cheng J-T. The use of herbal medicine in cancer-related anorexia/ cachexia treatment around the world. Curr Pharm Des 2012;18:4819-26.
18. Ohwada S, Satoh Y, Kawate S, Yamada T, Kawamura O, Koyama T et al. Low-Dose Erythromycin Reduces Delayed Gastric Emptying

and Improves Gastric Motility After Billroth I Pylorus-Preserving Pancreaticoduodenectomy. Ann Surg 2001;234:668-74.
19. McMillan DC. The systemic inflammation-based Glasgow Prognostic Score: a decade of experience in patients with cancer. Cancer Treat Rev 2013;39:534-40.
20. Lundholm K, Gelin J, Hyltander A, Lönnroth C, Sandström R, Svaninger G et al. Anti-inflammatory treatment may prolong survival in undernourished patients with metastatic solid tumors. Cancer Res 1994;54:5602-6.
21. Wigmore SJ, Falconer JS, Plester CE, Ross JA, Maingay JP, Carter DC et al. Ibuprofen reduces energy expenditure and acute-phase protein production compared with placebo in pancreatic cancer patients. Br J Cancer 1995;72:185-8.
22. Mantovani G, Macciò A, Madeddu C, Gramignano G, Serpe R, Massa E et al. Randomized phase III clinical trial of five different arms of treatment for patients with cancer cachexia: interim results. Nutrition 2008;24:305-13.
23. Solheim TS, Fearon KCH, Blum D, Kaasa S. Non-steroidal anti-inflammatory treatment in cancer cachexia: a systematic literature review. Acta Oncol 2013;52:6-17.
24. Dewey A, Baughan C, Dean T, Higgins B, Johnson I. Eicosapentaenoic acid (EPA, an omega-3 fatty acid from fish oils) for the treatment of cancer cachexia. Cochrane Database Syst Rev 2007;CD004597.
25. Colomer R, Moreno-Nogueira JM, García-Luna PP, García-Peris P, García-de-Lorenzo A, Zarazaga A et al. N-3 fatty acids, cancer and cachexia: a systematic review of the literature. Br J Nutr 2007;97:823-31.
26. van der Meij BS, Langius JA, Smit EF, Spreeuwenberg MD, von Blomberg BM, Heijboer AC et al. Oral nutritional supplements containing (n-3) polyunsaturated fatty acids affect the nutritional status of patients with stage III non-small cell lung cancer during multimodality treatment. J Nutr 2010;140:1774-80.
27. Murphy RA, Mourtzakis M, Chu QSC, Baracos VE, Reiman T, Mazurak VC. Nutritional intervention with fish oil provides a benefit over standard of care for weight and skeletal muscle mass in patients with nonsmall cell lung cancer receiving chemotherapy. Cancer 2011;117:1775-82.
28. Murphy RA, Mourtzakis M, Chu QS, Baracos VE, Reiman T, Mazurak VC. Supplementation with fish oil increases first-line chemotherapy efficacy in patients with advanced nonsmall cell lung cancer. Cancer 2011;117:3774-80.
29. Bayliss TJ, Smith JT, Schuster M, Dragnev KH, Rigas JR. A humanized anti-IL-6 antibody (ALD518) in non-small cell lung cancer. Expert Opin Biol Ther 2011;11:1663-8.
30. Ando K, Takahashi F, Motojima S, Nakashima K, Kaneko N, Hoshi K et al. Possible role for tocilizumab, an anti-interleukin-6 receptor antibody, in treating cancer cachexia. J Clin Oncol 2013;31:e69-72.
31. Hirata H, Tetsumoto S, Kijima T, Kida H, Kumagai T, Takahashi R et al. Favorable responses to tocilizumab in two patients with cancer-related cachexia. J Pain Symptom Manage 2013; 46:e9-e13.
32. Espat NJ, Moldawer LL, Copeland EM. Cytokine-mediated alterations in host metabolism prevent nutritional repletion in cachectic cancer patients. J Surg Oncol 1995;58:77-82.
33. Moldawer LL, Copeland EM. Proinflammatory cytokines, nutritional support, and the cachexia syndrome: interactions and therapeutic options. Cancer 1997;79:1828-39.
34. Deans C, Wigmore SJ. Systemic inflammation, cachexia and prognosis in patients with cancer. Curr Opin Clin Nutr Metab Care 2005;8: 265-9.
35. Wiedenmann B, Malfertheiner P, Friess H, Ritch P, Arseneau J, Mantovani G et al. A multicenter, phase II study of infliximab plus gemcitabine in pancreatic cancer cachexia. J Support Oncol 2008; 6:18-25.
36. Jatoi A, Dakhil SR, Nguyen PL, Sloan JA, Kugler JW, Rowland KM et al. A placebo-controlled double blind trial of etanercept for the cancer anorexia/weight loss syndrome: results from N00C1 from the North Central Cancer Treatment Group. Cancer 2007;110:1396-403.
37. Goldberg RM, Loprinzi CL, Mailliard JA, O'Fallon JR, Krook JE, Ghosh C et al. Pentoxifylline for treatment of cancer anorexia and cachexia? A randomized, double-blind, placebo-controlled trial. J Clin Oncol 1995;13:2856-9.
38. Reid J, Mills M, Cantwell M, Cardwell CR, Murray LJ, Donnelly M. Thalidomide for managing cancer cachexia. Cochrane Database Syst Rev 2012;4:CD008664.
39. Lundholm K, Körner U, Gunnebo L, Sixt-Ammilon P, Fouladiun M, Daneryd P et al. Insulin treatment in cancer cachexia: effects on surviv-

al, metabolism, and physical functioning. Clin Cancer Res 2007;13:2699-706.
40. Wang W, Iresjö BM, Karlsson L, Svanberg E. Provision of rhIGF-I/IGFBP-3 complex attenuated development of cancer cachexia in an experimental tumor model. Clin Nutr 2000;9:127-32.
41. Sridhar SS, Goodwin PJ. Insulin-insulin-like growth factor axis and colon cancer. J Clin Oncol 2009;27:165-7.
42. Chlebowski RT, Herrold J, Ali I, Oktay E, Chlebowski JS, Ponce AT et al. Influence of nandrolone decanoate on weight loss in advanced non-small cell lung cancer. Cancer 1986;58:183-6.
43. Zilbermint MF, Dobs AS. Nonsteroidal selective androgen receptor modulator Ostarine in cancer cachexia. Future Oncol 2009;5:1211-20.
44. Costelli P, Muscaritoli M, Bonetto A, Penna F, Reffo P, Bossola M et al. Muscle myostatin signalling is enhanced in experimental cancer cachexia. Eur J Clin Invest 2008;38:531-8.
45. Prado CM, Bekaii-Saab T, Doyle LA, Shrestha S, Ghosh S, Baracos VE et al. Skeletal muscle anabolism is a side effect of therapy with the MEK inhibitor: selumetinib in patients with cholangiocarcinoma. Br J Cancer 2012; 106:1583-6.
46. Carbó N, López-Soriano J, Costelli P, Busquets S, Alvarez B, Baccino FM et al. Interleukin-15 antagonizes muscle protein waste in tumour-bearing rats. Br J Cancer 2000;83:526-31.
47. Stofkova A. Cachexia - The interplay between the immune system, brain control and metabolism [Internet]. In: Khatami M, editor. Inflammatory Diseases - Immunopathology, Clinical and Pharmacological Bases. Rijeka, Croatia: InTech; 2012. p. 27-56. Available from: www.intechopen.com
48. Jatoi A, Alberts SR, Foster N, Morton R, Burch P, Block M et al. Is bortezomib, a proteasome inhibitor, effective in treating cancer-associated weight loss? Preliminary results from the North Central Cancer Treatment Group. Support Care Cancer 2005;13:381-6.
49. Joassard OR, Durieux A-C, Freyssenet DG. β2-Adrenergic agonists and the treatment of skeletal muscle wasting disorders. Int J Biochem Cell Biol 2013;45:2309-21.
50. Hyltander A, Daneryd P, Sandström R, Körner U, Lundholm K. Beta-adrenoceptor activity and resting energy metabolism in weight losing cancer patients. Eur J Cancer 2000;36: 330-4.
51. Busquets S, Figueras MT, Fuster G, Almendro V, Moore-Carrasco R, Ametller E et al. Anticachectic effects of formoterol: a drug for potential treatment of muscle wasting. Cancer Res 2004;64:6725-31.
52. Greig CA, Johns N, Gray C, MacDonald A, Stephens NA, Skipworth RJ et al. Phase I/II trial of formoterol fumarate combined with megestrol acetate in cachectic patients with advanced malignancy. Support Care Cancer 2014;22:1269-75.
53. Gold J. Proposed treatment of cancer by inhibition of gluconeogenesis. Oncology 1968; 22:185-207.
54. Loprinzi CL, Kuross SA, O'Fallon JR, Gesme DH, Gerstner JB, Rospond RM et al. Randomized placebo-controlled evaluation of hydrazine sulfate in patients with advanced colorectal cancer. J Clin Oncol 1994;12:1121-5.
55. Loprinzi CL, Goldberg RM, Su JQ, Mailliard JA, Kuross SA, Maksymiuk AW et al. Placebo-controlled trial of hydrazine sulfate in patients with newly diagnosed non-small-cell lung cancer. J Clin Oncol 1994;12:1126-9.
56. Agteresch HJ, Dagnelie PC, van der Gaast A, Stijnen T, Wilson JH. Randomized clinical trial of adenosine 5'-triphosphate in patients with advanced non-small-cell lung cancer. J Natl Cancer Inst 2000;92:321-8.
57. Beijer S, Hupperets PS, van den Borne BE, Eussen SR, van Henten AM, van den Beuken-van Everdingen M et al. Effect of adenosine 5'-triphosphate infusions on the nutritional status and survival of preterminal cancer patients. Anticancer Drugs 2009;20:625-33.
58. Beijer S, Hupperets PS, van den Borne BEEM, Wijckmans NEG, Spreeuwenberg C, van den Brandt PA et al. Randomized clinical trial on the effects of adenosine 5'-triphosphate infusions on quality of life, functional status, and fatigue in preterminal cancer patients. J Pain Symptom Manage 2010;40:520-30.
59. Chlebowski RT, Bulcavage L, Grosvenor M, Oktay E, Block JB, Chlebowski JS et al. Hydrazine sulfate influence on nutritional status and survival in non-small-cell lung cancer. J. Clin. Oncol 1990;8:9-15.

NUTRACEUTICALS IN CANCER PATIENTS WITH CACHEXIA

A. MOLFINO, G. GIOIA

INTRODUCTION

A nutraceutical is a product purified or isolated from food, often commercially available in medicinal form not associated with food and that has proved to present or enhance physiological benefits or to determine protection against pathological conditions.[1] The dietary supplement industry considers nutraceuticals as any non-toxic food component with scientifically proven health benefits in the prevention and/or treatment of a disease.[2] The term "nutraceutical", coming from "nutrition" and "pharmaceutical", was coined in 1989 by the chairman of the Foundation for Innovation in Medicine, an American medical health organization.[3,4] Nutraceuticals may increase the health value of diet, may enhance longer life, may reduce the development of health problems and may have a psychological benefit, as also perceived to be more "natural" than traditional medicine, and may result in fewer side effects.[5] We can classify nutraceuticals as potential nutraceuticals and established nutraceuticals. A potential nutraceutical has the promise of medical benefits and becomes established after sufficient evidences of its efficacy has been collected.[2] Nutraceuticals can be categorized as probiotics, prebiotics, dietary fibers, omega-3 fatty acids (ω-3 FAs) and antioxidants.[6] Market trends in nutraceuticals include functional foods, dietary supplements, and herbal/natural products.[2]

In this chapter we analyze the most important nutraceutical compounds belonging to the category of dietary supplements and their possible use in cancer cachexia, also describing their metabolic and molecular effects. In particular, we analyze those nutraceuticals which demonstrated the most efficacy in the treatment of cancer cachexia, *i.e.* ω-3 FAs, carnitine, β-hydroxy-β-methylbutyrate (HMB), branched-chain amino acids (BCAAs), and other amino acids (Fig. 6.1). Cancer cachexia is not reversed by standard nutritional support since it results from the combination of anorexia, reduced food intake and metabolic changes which lead to increased catabolism and the onset of anabolic resistance.[7]

The interest in the cancer-preventing/therapeutic property of the nutraceuticals is based on their ability to affect multiple deranged signaling pathways in cancer cells, including epigenetic regulation. Nutraceuticals are increasingly noted to alter microRNAs/cancer stem cells expression and function but the molecular mechanisms are not yet clearly identified.[8]

OMEGA-3 FATTY ACIDS

The anti-inflammatory effects of ω-3 FAs, present in large amounts in fish oil, may be beneficial in the prevention and treatment of cancer cachexia, considering that inflammatory cytokines play a significant role in the pathogenesis of cancer cachexia.[9] Larger randomized controlled trials mostly did not find a significant effect of ω-3 FAs supplementation in advanced cachectic cancer patients while smaller trials reported positive effects.[10] Oral supplementation of ω-3 FAs in cancer patients during chemo-radiotherapy and in

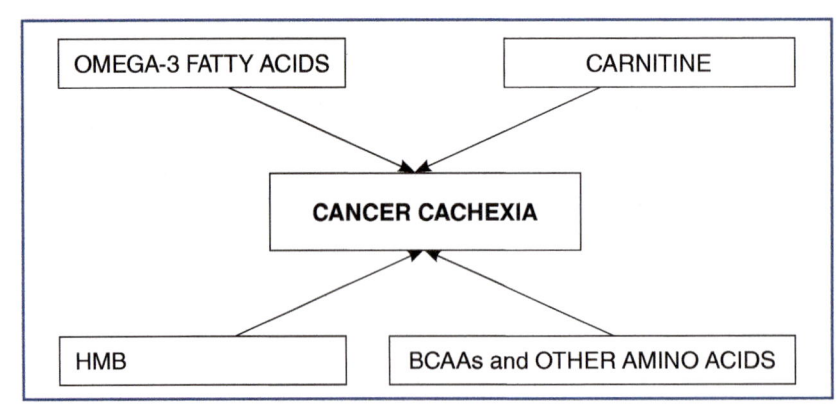

Figure 6.1 – The main nutraceuticals used in the treatment of cancer cachexia [β-hydroxy-β-methylbutyrate (HMB), branched-chain amino acids (BCAAs)].

palliative care beneficially affects quality of life and body weight, with no effects on Karnofsky performance status and survival.[11] Eicosapentaenoic acid (EPA)-enriched oral nutritional supplementation for five weeks in 40 lung cancer patients receiving multimodal treatment improved quality of life and functional status.[12] In another study, 40 lung cancer patients receiving chemotherapy were supplemented with fish oil [2.5 g EPA + docosaexaenoic acid (DHA)/day] for 10 weeks maintaining their weight whereas a control group of patients experienced significant weight loss. Muscle mass was maintained or gained in the supplemented group compared to the control patients.[13] EPA-enriched oral nutritional perioperative supplementation in head and neck cancer patients was associated with amelioration in lean body mass but the limited relevance of this study is due to the lack of a control group.[14] Recent evidence, confirmed by a post hoc dose-response analysis, indicates that protein and energy dense ω-3-FA-enriched oral supplementation (≥2.2 g EPA/day) improves lean body mass and quality of life in cachectic patients with advanced pancreatic cancer.[15] ω-3 polyunsaturated fatty acids (PUFAs) have been noted to reduce not only tissue wasting but also tumor growth.[16,17] Conversely, a meta-analysis reported no effect of EPA on cachexia in advanced cancer patients, comparing EPA combined with protein energy supplementation versus protein energy supplementation alone.[18] A large multicenter trial indicated that EPA alone is not successful in the treatment of weight-losing patients with advanced gastrointestinal or lung cancer.[19]

CARNITINE

L-Carnitine, a vitamin-like amino acid derivative, is an essential factor involved in FA metabolism as an acyltransferase cofactor and in energy production processes, such as interconversion in the mechanisms of regulation of ketogenesis and thermogenesis. The endogenous carnitine pool is maintained by biosynthesis and absorption of carnitine from the diet. Carnitine has one asymmetric carbon giving two stereoisomers (D and L), but only L-carnitine has biological effects. Stressful conditions or diseases may significantly lower the endogenous liver synthesis of carnitine. The carnivorous human diet is very high in carnitine, while the herbivore diet is very low.[20] Although the human body can synthesize L-carnitine, about 80% of this compound is delivered by food. Animal by-products contain the highest amount of L-carnitine, such as beef and milk products. L-carnitine is very low in vegetables, fruits, lipids, sunflower oil. Mushrooms present high levels of L-carnitine.[21] Carnitine is present in cardiac and skeletal muscle and is involved in the utilization of FAs for energy in the muscle cells, probably being glycogen sparing and reducing lactic acid production, thus improving muscle function and endurance. Human studies have not shown an increase in muscle carnitine or improvement in performance in healthy individuals from carnitine supplementation but an improvement was seen in heart and skeletal muscle performances in humans with impaired oxygen supply.[22] Administration of 1 g/kg body weight of L-carnitine to highly cachectic rats bearing the AH-130 Yoshida ascites hepatoma results in a significant improvement in food intake, muscle weight, and physical performance. L-carnitine administration significantly decreases proteolytic rate by reducing proteasome activity and the gene expression of ubiquitin, C8 proteasome subunit, MuRF-1, and caspase-3.[23] Chronic systemic inflammation and increased oxidative stress contributes to the cancer cachexia syndrome. Carnitine may represent a further therapeutic tool against cachexia because carnitine supplementation has been shown to reduce chronic inflammation, oxidative stress and fatigue in cancer patients, but more studies are necessary to recommend its clinical use.[24] Seventy-two advanced pancreatic cancer patients received orally 4 g of L-Carnitine for 12 weeks with a significant improvement in body mass index. Body cell mass, body fat and quality of life also improved after L-Carnitine supplementation. A trend was observed towards an increase in overall survival and towards a decrease in hospital stay. Pancreatic cancer patients may benefit from L-Carnitine supplementation.[25]

β-HYDROXY-β-METHYLBUTYRATE

Administration of the leucine metabolite HMB could be a viable component in multimodal therapies targeting cancer cachexia. HMB treatment promotes myogenesis, suppresses protein degradation, and activates protein synthesis and skeletal muscle growth and preservation.[26] In an experimental model of cancer cachexia, Wistar rats were randomized to receive standard or 4% HMB-enriched chow. The growth of the AH-130 ascites hepatoma induced significant carcass weight and gastrocnemius muscle loss. In HMB-treated tumor-bearing rats, body weight was not lost but significantly increased, and gastrocnemius loss was significantly attenuated. HMB increased the phosphorylation of key anabolic molecules thus suggesting an improved muscle protein anabolism.[27] Several studies support HMB efficacy in preventing exercise-related muscle damage in healthy trained and untrained individuals as well as muscle loss during chronic diseases. The dosage of 3 g/day may be routinely recommended to maintain or improve muscle mass, and consequently function within an unequivocal safety profile of HMB but further clinical studies are needed to confirm its effectiveness in pathological conditions.[28] Thirty-two advanced cancer patients supplemented with HMB/Arginine/Glutamine gained body mass after four weeks. This gain derived from a significant increase in fat-free mass that was maintained over the 24 weeks.

This effect could be attributed to the capacity of HMB to reduce protein breakdown and improve protein synthesis in combination with arginine and glutamine.[29] Cachectic loss of muscle mass can be opposed by HMB with other compounds in a complex core nutraceutical program.[30]

BRANCHED-CHAIN AMINO ACIDS AND OTHER AMINO ACIDS

The BCAAs leucine and valine significantly suppressed the loss of body weight in MAC16 tumor-bearing mice, producing a significant increase in skeletal muscle wet weight, through an increase in protein synthesis and a decrease in protein degradation.[31] BCAAs as the protein component of total parenteral nutrition (TPN) were administered to malnourished patients with intra-abdominal adenocarcinoma. Leucine and tyrosine flux increased significantly. Leucine oxidation was significantly higher while tyrosine oxidation was significantly lower thus suggesting improved protein utilization. Whole body protein synthesis and breakdown were significantly higher on BCAA-TPN using the tyrosine tracer. When using the leucine tracers synthesis and breakdown were not significantly increased. The fractional albumin synthetic rate in particular increased significantly on BCAA-TPN.[32] Similar effects were described in a small group of malnourished cancer patients with intra-abdominal metastatic adenocarcinoma receiving BCAA-enriched TPN formula containing 50% of the amino acids as BCAAs. An increase in whole body leucine flux and oxidation, an increase in protein synthesis were shown, and leucine incorporation was significantly increased. BCAA-enriched formulas improve whole body leucine kinetics and albumin synthesis, thus favorably influencing protein metabolism in cachectic patients.[33] TPN for two weeks was superior to oral and enteral feeding in increasing plasma amino acid levels in patients with esophageal cancer.[34] High provision of amino acids, with consequent hyperaminoacidemia, is able to stimulate the anabolic protein response in non-small cell lung cancer patients with moderate cachexia and considerable resistance of whole-body protein anabolism.[35] Infusion of 2 g amino acid/kg/day, with high doses of BCAAs, ameliorates protein metabolism of severely malnourished cancer patients. International guidelines based on larger randomized trials are needed to indicate the optimal dosage of BCAAs and other amino acids in cancer cachexia.[36]

CONCLUSIONS

Analysis of the most consistent data available allows us to indicate that nutraceuticals are key factors in the treatment of cancer cachexia. Certainly, more clinical trials are required to routinely use nutraceuticals in clinical practice. The lack of regulation of these products represents a limit for researchers and physicians in order to establish correct experimental protocols to test and confirm the efficacy and safety of nutraceuticals.

REFERENCES

1. Bull E. What is nutraceutical? Pharm J 2000; 265:57-8.
2. De Felice L Stephen. The nutraceutical revolution, its impact on food industry. Trends in Food Sci and Tech 1995;6:59-61.
3. Mannion M. Nutraceutical revolution continues at foundation for innovation in medicine conference. Am J Nat Med 1998;5:30-3.
4. Dureja D, Kaushik D, Kumar V. Developments in nutraceuticals. Indian J Pharmacol 2003;35: 363-72.
5. Manisha P, Rohit K V, Shubhini AS. Nutraceuticals: new era of medicine and health. Asian J Pharm Clin Res 2010;3:11-5.
6. Kokate CK, Purohit AP, Gokhale SB. Nutraceutical and Cosmaceutical. Pharmacognosy, 21st edition. Pune, India: Nirali Prakashan; 2002. p. 542-9.
7. Fearon K, Strasser F, Anker SD, Bosaeus I, Bruera E, Fainsinger RL *et al*. Definition and classification of cancer cachexia: an international consensus. Lancet Oncol 2011;12:489-95.
8. Ahmad A, Li Y, Bao B, Kong D, Sarkar FH. Epigenetic regulation of miRNA-cancer stem cells nexus by nutraceuticals. Mol Nutr Food Res 2014;58:79-86.
9. Seruga B, Zhang H, Bernstein LJ, Tannock IF. Cytokines and their relationship to the symptoms and outcome of cancer. Nat Rev Cancer 2008;8:887-99.
10. Ries A, Trottenberg P, Elsner F *et al*. A systematic review on the role of fish oil for the treatment of cachexia in advanced cancer: an EPCRC cachexia guidelines project. Palliat Med 2012;26:294-304.
11. van der Meij BS, van Bokhorst-de van der Schueren MA, Langius JA, Brouwer IA, van Leeuwen PA. n-3 PUFAs in cancer, surgery, and critical care: a systematic review on clinical

11. effects, incorporation, and washout of oral or enteral compared with parenteral supplementation. Am J Clin Nutr 2011;94:1248-65.
12. van der Meij BS, Langius JA, Spreeuwenberg MD, Slootmaker SM, Paul MA, Smit EF et al. Oral nutritional supplements containing n-3 polyunsaturated fatty acids affect quality of life and functional status in lung cancer patients during multimodality treatment: an RCT. Eur J Clin Nutr 2012;66:399-404.
13. Murphy RA, Mourtzakis M, Chu QS, Baracos VE, Reiman T, Mazurak VC et al. Nutritional intervention with fish oil provides a benefit over standard of care for weight and skeletal muscle mass in patients with nonsmall cell lung cancer receiving chemotherapy. Cancer 2011;117: 1775-82.
14. Weed HG, Ferguson ML, Gaff RL et al. Lean body mass gain in patients with head and neck squamous cell cancer treated perioperatively with a protein and energy-dense nutritional supplement containing eicosapentaenoic acid. Head Neck 2011;33:1027-33.
15. Fearon KC, Von Meyenfeldt MF, Moses AG, Van Geenen R, Roy A, Gouma DJ,et al. Effect of a protein and energy dense N-3 fatty acid enriched oral supplement on loss of weight and lean tissue in cancer cachexia: a randomised double blind trial. Gut 2003;52:1479e86.
16. Rose DP, Connolly JM. Effects of dietary omega-3 fatty acids on human breast cancer growth and metastases in nude mice. J Natl Cancer Inst 1993;85:1743e7.
17. Tisdale MJ. Mechanism of lipid mobilization associated with cancer cachexia: interaction between the polyunsaturated fatty acid, eicosapentaenoic acid, and inhibitory guanine nucleotide-regulatory protein. Prostaglandins Leukot Essent Fatty Acids 1993;48: 105e9.
18. Dewey A, Baughan C, Dean T, Higgins B, Johnson I et al. Eicosapentaenoic acid (EPA, an omega-3 fatty acid from fish oils) for the treatment of cancer cachexia. Cochrane Database Syst Rev 2007:CD004597.
19. Fearon KC, Barber MD, Moses AG, Ahmedzai SH, Taylor GS, Tisdale MJ et al. Double-blind, placebo-controlled, randomized study of eicosapentaenoic acid diester in patients with cancer cachexia. J Clin Oncol 2006;24:3401e7.
20. Dąbrowska M, Starek M. Analytical approaches to determination of carnitine in biological materials, foods and dietary supplements. Food Chem 2014;142:220-32.
21. Rospond B, Chłopicka J. The biological function of L-carnitine and its content in the particular food examples. Przegl Lek 2013;70:85-91.
22. Cerretelli P, Marconi C. L-carnitine supplementation in humans. The effects of physical performance. J Sports Med 1990;11:1-14.
23. Busquets S, Serpe R, Toledo M, Betancourt A, Marmonti E, Orpí M et al. L-Carnitine: an adequate supplement for a multi-targeted anti-wasting therapy in cancer. Clin Nutr 2012; 31:889-95.
24. Laviano A, Meguid MM, Guijarro A, Muscaritoli M, Cascino A, Preziosa I et al. Antimyopathic effects of carnitine and nicotine. Curr Opin Clin Nutr Metab Care 2006;9:442-8.
25. Kraft M, Kraft K, Gärtner S, Mayerle J, Simon P, Weber E et al. L-Carnitine-supplementation in advanced pancreatic cancer (CARPAN)- a randomized multicentre trial. Nutr J 2012;11:52.
26. Kim JS, Khamoui AV, Jo E et al. β-Hydroxy-β-methylbutyrate as a countermeasure for cancer cachexia: a cellular and molecular rationale. Anticancer Agents Med Chem 2013;13: 1188-96.
27. Aversa Z, Bonetto A, Costelli P, Minero VG, Penna F, Baccino FM et al. β-hydroxy-β-methylbutyrate (HMB) attenuates muscle and body weight loss in experimental cancer cachexia. Int J Oncol 2011;38:713-20.
28. Molfino A, Gioia G, Rossi Fanelli F et al. Beta-hydroxy-beta-methylbutyrate supplementation in health and disease: a systematic review of randomized trials. Amino Acids 2013;45: 1273-92.
29. May PE, Barber A, D'Olimpio JT, Hourihane A, Abumrad NN. Reversal of cancer-related wasting using oral supplementation with a combination of beta-hydroxy-beta-methylbutyrate, arginine, and glutamine. Am J Surg 2002;183:471-9.
30. McCarty MF, Block KI. Toward a core nutraceutical program for cancer management. Integr Cancer Ther 2006;5:150-71.
31. Eley HL, Russell ST, Tisdale MJ. Effect of branched-chain amino acids on muscle atrophy in cancer cachexia. Biochem J 2007;407: 113-20.
32. Hunter DC, Weintraub M, Blackburn GL, Bis-

trian BR. Branched chain amino acids as the protein component of parenteral nutrition in cancer cachexia. Br J Surg 1989;76:149-53.

33. Tayek JA, Bistrian BR, Hehir DJ, Martin R, Moldawer LL, Blackburn GL *et al*. Improved protein kinetics and albumin synthesis by branched chain amino acid-enriched total parenteral nutrition in cancer cachexia. A prospective randomized crossover trial. Cancer 1986;58:147-57.

34. Pearlstone DB, Lee JI, Alexander RH, Chang TH, Brennan MF, Burt M. Effect of enteral and parenteral nutrition on amino acid levels in cancer patients. JPEN J Parenter Enteral Nutr 1995;19:204-8.

35. Winter A, MacAdams J, Chevalier S. Normal protein anabolic response to hyperaminoacidemia in insulin-resistant patients with lung cancer cachexia. Clin Nutr 2012;31:765-73.

36. Bozzetti F, Bozzetti V. Is the intravenous supplementation of amino acid to cancer patients adequate? A critical appraisal of literature. Clin Nutr 2013;32:142-6.

PERSPECTIVES

F. ROSSI FANELLI

Significant progress has been achieved in recent years regarding the re-definition and classification of cachexia in cancer.[1,2] Despite its detrimental consequences for the prognosis and quality of life of cancer patients, however, cancer cachexia is still poorly recognized, prevented and treated.[3] As a consequence, up to one in five cancer patients still dies because of the direct effects of cachexia.[4] While the incidence of some tumors is slowly decreasing, the prevalence of cancer is steadily increasing, due to the progress achieved in early cancer diagnosis and treatment. The population of cancer survivors is expanding worldwide, with the "cancer journey" progressively becoming a long-term experience in which the burden of comorbidities negatively affects both patient health and the efficacy of healthcare systems. In a such clinical scenario, cachexia is a significantly prevalent condition of cancer impacting negatively on numerous outcomes. Several efforts have been made in order to reduce such prognostic impact, although more work must be done, particularly in translating molecular and experimental findings into clinical practice.[5]

Over the past 10 years, our understanding of the biology and molecular mechanisms of cancer cachexia has considerably expanded, and several new pathways involved in its pathophysiology have been discovered. According to novel pathophysiological knowledge, new cachexia therapies have been implemented, mainly aimed at acting on specific molecular targets such as myostatin, ghrelin, interleukin-6, interleukin-1α, and skeletal muscle androgen receptors.[5] Translational medicine has proved to be productive in the cancer cachexia field, however no single agent is able alone to counteract this devastating syndrome. A practical biomarker able to directly identify cancer patients predisposed to developing cachexia is currently lacking. Clinical signs, together with laboratory findings (*i.e.* inflammatory markers), help physicians to identify such vulnerable patients. Practically all patients affected by cancer undergo an additional risk of developing cachexia and several metabolic changes can be detected even with minimal body composition alterations. An accurate assessment associated with a recurring follow-up should be implemented in parallel with oncological monitoring in order to promote an early diagnosis and a prompt efficacious intervention as well.[6] Skeletal muscle, contributing to more than 40% of body weight, seems to be the main tissue involved in the wasting that takes place during cancer cachexia, however recent developments suggest that tissues and organs such as adipose tissue (both BAT and WAT), brain, liver, gut and heart are directly involved in the cachectic process and may be connected to muscle wasting.[4] Cancer cachexia can be considered a multi-organ syndrome, and effective therapy should be therefore based on multimodal intervention.[7] Such an approach includes gradual resistance training, aerobic exercise, targeted nutrient supplementation and pharmacological intervention and currently represents the best available modality with which to face cancer cachexia, although it is not yet evidence-based. More research and more clinical trials are necessary in order to better define the impact of this tailored intervention for cancer cachexia. The scientific community should, however, direct their attention into broadening the horizons of this topic: fighting cancer cachexia should include an integrated approach based on a multilevel intervention strategy operating in different domains: Teaching, Awareness, Recognition, Genetics, Exercise/Early Intervention and Treatment of cancer cachexia (the T.A.R.G.E.T. approach).[7] Evidence of cancer cachexia's impact on patient outcomes is now enough that it is not possibly to justify its underestimation and unmet medical needs. What we really need is a multimodal strategy (such as the T.A.R.G.E.T. approach) that promotes awareness of cancer cachexia, making it in turn more recognizable and properly treatable.

REFERENCES

1. Fearon K, Strasser F, Anker SD *et al*. Definition and classification of cancer cachexia: an international consensus. Lancet Oncol 2011;12: 489-95.

2. Muscaritoli M, Anker SD, Argiles J, Aversa Z, Bauer JM, Biolo G *et al*. Consensus definition of sarcopenia, cachexia and pre-cachexia: joint document elaborated by Special Interest Groups (SIG) "cachexia-anorexia in chronic wasting diseases" and "nutrition in geriatrics." Clin Nutr 2010;29:154-9.

3. von Haehling S, Anker SD. Prevalence, incidence and clinical impact of cachexia: facts and numbers-update 2014. J Cachexia Sarcopenia Muscle 2014;5:261-3.

4. Vaughan VC, Martin P, Lewandowski PA. Cancer cachexia: impact, mechanisms and emerging treatments. J Cachexia Sarcopenia Muscle 2013;4:95-109.

5. von Haehling S, Anker SD. Treatment of Cachexia: An Overview of Recent Developments. J Am Med Dir Assoc 2014;15:866-72.

6. Muscaritoli M, Molfino A, Gioia G, Laviano A, Rossi Fanelli F. The "parallel pathway": a novel nutritional and metabolic approach to cancer patients. Intern Emerg Med 2011;6:105-12.

7. Muscaritoli M, Molfino A, Lucia S, Rossi Fanelli F. Cachexia: A preventable comorbidity of cancer. A T.A.R.G.E.T. approach. Crit Rev Oncol/Hematol (2014), http://dx.doi.org/10.1016/j.critrevonc.2014.10.014

PRINTED BY
EDIZIONI MINERVA MEDICA
MAY 2015
SALUZZO (ITALY)
CORSO IV NOVEMBRE, 29-31

NOTES

NOTES

NOTES

NOTES

NOTES

NOTES

NOTES